neurofibrillary of the brain, causing oxidative stress, excessive chronic inflammation, and further mitochondrial dysfunction. It is a vicious cycle where the symptoms continuously cause the disease to worsen, which in turn makes the symptoms also worsen.

The many components of Alzheimer's disease lead to the brain's neurons becoming insulin resistant, and when they are no longer able to absorb the glucose needed, they can also no longer fuel the cells, leading to cellular starvation and death. But, as intermittent fasting repairs mitochondrial cells and increases them in number, it can also increase the number of cells able to fuel off of non-glucose fuels. Additionally, intermittent fasting can treat the insulin resistance itself and cause the production of ketones to fuel the non-mitochondrial neural cells.

Cancer

Intermittent fasting has been known to be of several benefits to the human body, one of which is the prevention of cancer. Studies have found that intermittent fasting can reduce your likelihood of developing cancer and help make cancer treatment more successful. Intermittent fasting works to help tackle several other health risks that are in turn factors for the development of cancer. Conditions like diabetes, obesity, etc., are linked to the rise in cancer cases. Intermittent fasting helps tackle these which, in turn, help protect us against cancer. Another important reason for seeing intermittent fasting as beneficial to cancer prevention and treatment could be because fasting helps regulate blood sugar. Fasting triggers stem cells to produce more and more immune-boosting cells as well as tumor-killing cells. With the help of balanced nutritional intake, precursors to cancer are held in check by following an intermittent fasting schedule.

Studies on mice and other animals also showed how intermittent fasting could help produce better outcomes of chemotherapy in the treatment of cancer. Reduction of toxicity was another important observation after following intermittent fasting, which is valuable in cancer treatments.

Why Does Intermittent Fasting Affects Women's Hormones More Than Men's?

If you have been doing research online, then you might have read claims such as "intermittent fasting is not for women" or "if women intermittent fast, their hormones will be out of whack." Which isn't the case. We will discuss how intermittent fasting truly affects women's hormone as when compared to men's.

To briefly talk about men, they were created to "hunt and gather" so to speak. Unlike women, they do not have to carry a baby, which is one of the reasons why intermittent fasting does not affect men as drastically as it does women.

Women tend to trigger these hormones differently when compared to men, and the main problem occurs because of kisspeptin. For readers that don't know what kisspeptin is, it is a protein-like molecule that neurons use to communicate with each other. Women tend to produce more kisspeptin when compared to men, which is a precursor to a Gonadotropin-releasing hormone (GnRH).

Also, scientists noticed that female rats' luteinizing hormone plummeted as their estrogen levels went thru the roof. To briefly touch upon thyroid, t3 levels were deceased. However, t3 levels are always decreasing between meals. The t4, which is responsible for producing thyroid, remained the same. This means the thyroid isn't being affected drastically. It is always suggested that you get regular blood work done to ensure your thyroid is fine.

If you feel cold all the time, then the chances are your thyroid levels are lower. If you notice that you are getting to starve throughout the day, and it becomes tough to fast, then break the fast and try it again at a later date. As women, you need to listen to your body more than men, as women tend to be more sensitive to hormones when intermittent fasting.

Changes in Your Body After Age 50

If you have reached age fifty, then you should congratulate yourself. You have been through school, adolescence, relationships, children, and most importantly, the changing of your body. You might be looking at your body and asking yourself exactly what happened to it during the last few years. Some things you may have not been able to control. Such as, hereditary medical issues and the ravage that time puts on our bodies. Accidents and illnesses are also beyond our control. But, you can now begin to understand the changes in your body and make plans to reduce or eliminate as many of the negative changes as you possibly can.

The first thing that will probably happen to you in your fifties is the onset of menopause. The most notable thing about menopause is that your monthly periods will stop – forever! Menopause is the biggest single change that your body will ever experience besides puberty. Menopause can lead to belly fat, weight gain, and osteoporosis. It is a natural occurrence in the life of every woman, caused by the body making less of the hormone's estrogen and progesterone.

Estrogens (there are more than one) is the name for the group of sex-related hormones that make women be women. They cause and promote the initial development and further maintenance of female characteristics in the human body. Estrogens are what give you breasts, hair in the right places, the ability to reproduce, and your monthly cycle. Estrogen is the hormone that does all of the long-term work in maintaining femininity. Progesterone has one purpose in the woman's body, and that is to implant the egg in the uterus and keep her pregnant until it is time to deliver the baby.

In women, estrogen is crucial to becoming and remaining womanly. In the ovaries, it stimulates the growth of eggs for reproduction. It causes the vagina to grow to proper adult size. Estrogen promotes the healthy growth of the fallopian tubes and the uterus. It also causes your breasts to grow and to fill with milk when a baby is coming. Estrogen is also responsible for making women store some excess fat around their thighs and hips. This weight storage is nature's way of ensuring that the baby will have nutrition during times of famine.

One of the forms of estrogen dramatically decreases in production after menopause, and this form helps women to regulate the rate of their metabolism and how fast they gain weight. After menopause women tend to gain more weight in their middle area of the body, in the abdomen. This fat collects around the organs and is known as visceral fat.

A lack of estrogen is not the only reason women tend to gain weight after age fifty. Besides a lack of estrogen, the biggest single reason that women over fifty gain weight is lifestyle changes. Small changes such as they are no longer running children to activities. Many women move less after fifty. Sometimes they move less because their joints have begun to ache. Stiffness begins to set in, especially in the morning, and rolling out of bed suddenly becomes a chore. Many continue to cook large meals and have difficulty scaling back to cooking for just one or two people, and someone needs to eat that extra food. Some women even feel that life ends when their children leave, so they might as well just indulge a little.

However, all of this indulging and relaxing leads to loss of muscle strength, loss of flexibility, and increased belly fat, which in turn leads to even more problems. This also leads to an increase in osteoporosis. The lack of estrogen is the leading cause of osteoporosis, which translates literally to the porous bone. The bones in the body, particularly the long bones of the arms and the legs, become more porous as the quality and density of the bone are reduced. Bones will continue to regrow and refresh themselves all of your life, but in osteoporosis, the bone is deteriorating faster than new growth can replace it.

Estrogen helps to decrease overall cholesterol levels in young women, which is why some women remain healthy even when they don't take the time to eat healthy meals. With all of these changes after the age of fifty, and post-menopause, suddenly estrogen levels can drop dramatically. This increase of cholesterol in the body can lead to strokes and heart attacks. Cholesterol is a substance that occurs naturally in your body and is made by the liver. Cholesterol in your body also comes from the foods that you eat.

HDL is the type of cholesterol known as the good type of cholesterol because it removes excess amounts of cholesterol from your arteries and then carries it to the liver where it can be metabolized and removed from the body during waste removal. LDL is the bad form of cholesterol because it likes to sit in your arteries and form deposits known as plaque. It is possible to have a high total cholesterol number and still be considered healthy if the number is high because the HDL is high and the LDL is low. This means that your body is doing the right thing and the good cholesterol is eliminating the bad cholesterol.

If you have gained a significant amount of weight your body will create new arteries to supply blood flow to this increased part of you. This will also make the heart work harder than it needs to. If plaque builds up in the arteries that are connected to the heart those arteries can become clogged which results in coronary artery disease. This can lead to a heart attack if a piece of plaque breaks loose and cuts off the steady flow of blood to the muscles of the heart.

Too much cholesterol has also been found in the brains of people who suffered from Alzheimer's disease. And an excessive amount of cholesterol can cause gallstones, which women are naturally at a higher risk of anyway.

You may have noticed that you seem to be losing control of your bladder function, or that laughing or sneezing makes you dribble a bit. This is also a normal effect of aging because the muscles are not as strong as they used to be. Also, the excess weight pressing down on the bladder does not help the situation.

While it is impossible to stop the process of aging there are things every woman can do to slow the process and help her body remain healthy far into the future. One of the most important ways women can do this is to maintain a healthy weight.

Types of intermittent fasting

There are so many different ways to practice intermittent fasting. This chapter is dedicated to the variety of these methods. I will walk you through 10 specific and different methods for IF before ending with a section on how to make your choice. By the end of this chapter, if you've chosen to try IF, you should feel that your IF plans have direction and form. Hopefully you will feel excited to implement these new plans into your daily routine.

Explanation of Different Methods

Before you can start practicing intermittent fasting and incorporating it into your lifestyle, you'll have to know all the possibilities so you can choose the right one(s) for yourself, your goals, your habits, and your body/personality type. Read through the following 10 suggestions to find which methods sound best for you.

Lean-Gains Method

The lean-gains method essentially focuses on the combined efforts of rigorous exercise, fasting, and a healthy diet. The fame surrounding this approach comes from its acclaimed success at turning fat directly into muscle. The goal is to fast within each day for 14-16 hours, starting when you wake up.

The ideal approach to the lean-gains method seems to be that you wake up and fast until 1 pm, doing some stretches and pre-workout warmups just before noon. Starting at noon, you would engage in training in whatever exercise you choose for an hour or less, ending with you breaking fast around 1 pm. Your meal at this time would be the largest of the day.

You would then engage in your day as normal past then, eating again around 4 pm, then eating for the final time around 9 pm, giving yourself a ~15-hour fast until the next day at 1 pm. If you choose this approach, yet feel a bit overwhelmed, you can work up to 15 hours, starting with a 13- or 14-hour fast for the first week, building up to 15- or 16-hour fasting after that.

16:8 Method

The 16:8 method is one of the most popular methods among Intermittent Fasters. You spend 16 hours within each day fasting, and the other 8 hours are your eating window. Most people try to choose their 8-hour eating window to be the times when they're primarily active. If you're a night person, feel free to make your eating window a little later. Hold off eating during the daytime as much as possible, then have breakfast around 3 or 4 pm. For morning people, have breakfast earlier, say, around 11 am, and stop food consumption by 7 pm.

16:8 is an incredibly flexible method that works for many different kinds of people. It is even flexible once you decide to try a particular fasting to eating window ratio. For example, if you don't seem to be jiving with the 11-7 pm eating window, you can absolutely alter the next day to suit your needs better. Maybe try waiting until later in the day to have breakfast! Try what you need to do, as long as you're keeping to that 16:8-hour ratio.

Whereas the lean-gains method technically applies the same hourly ratio, it's much more strict regarding healthy diet and exercise regimen. The 16:8 method does not need any type of exercise booster, but that's up to the practitioner. It is always best to try adding healthy dietary choices to one's IF eating schedule, but don't try to restrict too many calories, as it can incorporate to feelings of lightheadedness and low energy. With 16:8, you can eat what you need and swap the hours around as desired.

14:10 Method

Similar to the 16:8 method, the 14:10 method requires fasting and eating in varying degrees within each day. In this case, you would fast for 14 hours and engage in eating for a 10-hour window afterward. This method has the same flexibility as 16:8 in terms of what time of the day it's arranged around, and how easy it is to troubleshoot. Additionally, it is flexible in the sense that the eating window is two hours longer. This accommodates people with more intense physical routines or daily demands, as well as people who simply need to eat a little later in the day to feel well.

20:4 Method

Whereas the 14:10 method was an easier step down from 16:8 method, the 20:4 method is definitely a step up in terms of difficulty. It is certainly a more intense method, for it requires 20 hours of fasting within each day with only a 4-hour eating window for the individual to gain all his or her nutrients and energy.

Most people who try this method end up having either one large meal with several snacks or they have two smaller meals with fewer snacks. 20:4 is flexible in that sense—the sense whereby the individual chooses how the eating window is divided amongst meals and snacks.

The 20:4 method is tricky, many people instinctually over-eat during their eating window, but that's neither necessary nor is it healthy. People that choose the 20:4 method should try to keep meal portions around the same size that they would normally be without fasting. Experimenting on how many snacks are needed will be helpful as well with this method.

Many people work up to the 20:4 method from other methods, based on what their bodies can handle and what they're ready to attempt. Few start with 20:4, so if it's not working for you right away, please don't be too hard on yourself! Step it back to the 16:8 method and then see how soon you can get back to where you'd like to be.

The Warrior Method

The warrior method is quite similar to the 20:4 method in that the individual fasts for 20 hours within each day and breaks fast for a 4-hour eating window. The difference is in the outlook and mindset of the practitioner. The thought process behind the warrior method is that, in ancient times, the hunter coming home from stalking prey or the warrior coming home from battle would really only get one meal each day. One meal would have to provide sustenance for the rest of the day, recuperative energy from the ordeal, and sustainable energy for the future.

Therefore, practitioners of the warrior method are encouraged to have one large meal when they breakfast, and that meal should be jam-packed with fats, proteins, and carbs for the rest of the day (and for the days ahead). This is similar to the 20:4 method, however, it can sometimes be too intense for practitioners, and it's very easy to scale this one back in forcefulness by making up a method like 18:6 or 17:7. If it's not working, don't force it to work past two weeks, but do try to make it through a week to see if it's your stubbornness or if it's just a mismatch with the method.

12:12 Method

The 12:12 method is a little easier, along with the lines of the 14:10 method, rather than the 16:8 or 20:4 methods. Beginners to intermittent fasting would do well to try this one right off the bat. Some people get 12 hours of sleep each night and can easily wake up from the fasting period, ready to engage with the eating window. Many people use this method in their lives without even knowing it.

To go about the 12:12 method in your life, however, you'll want to be as purposeful about it as you can be. Make sure to be strict about your 12-hour cut-offs. Make sure it's working and feeling good in your body. Then you're invited to take things up a notch and try, say, 14:10 or maybe your own invention, like

15:11. As always, start with what works and then move up (or down) to what feels right (and even possibly better).

5:2 Method

The 5:2 method is popular among those who want to take things up a notch. Instead of fasting and eating within each day, these individuals take up a practice of fasting two whole days out of the week. The other 5 days are free to eat, exercise, or diet as desired. However, those other two days (which can be consecutive or scattered throughout the week) must be strictly fasting days.

However, for those fasting days, it's not as if the individual can't eat anything altogether. In actuality, one is allowed to consume no more than 500 calories each day for this intermittent fasting method. I suppose these fasting days would be better referred to as "restricted-intake" days, for that is a more accurate description.

The 5:2 method is extremely rewarding, but it is also one of the more difficult ones to attempt. If you're having issues with this method, don't be afraid to experiment the next week with a method like 14:10 or 16:8, where you're fasting and eating within each day. If that works better for you, don't be ashamed to embrace it! However, if you're dedicated to having days "on" and days "off" with fasting and eating, there are other alternatives, too.

Eat-Stop-Eat (24-Hour) Method

The eat-stop-eat, or 24-hour method, is another option for people who want to have days "on" and "off" between fasting and eating. It's a little less intense than the 5:2 method, and it's much more flexible for the individual, based on what he or she needs. For instance, if you just need a literal 24-hour fast each week, you can do that. On the other hand, if you want a more flexible method like the 5:2 method to happen, then you can work with what you want and create a method surrounding those desires and goals.

The most successful approaches to the eat-stop-eat method have involved more strict dieting (or at the very least, cautious and healthy eating) during the 5 or 6 days when the individual engages in the week's free-eating window. For the individual to truly see success with weight loss, there will have to be some caloric restriction (or high nutrition focus) during those 5 or 6 days, so that the body will have a version of consistency in health and nutrition content.

On the one or two days each week the individual decides to fast, there can still be highly-restricted caloric intake. As with the 5:2 method, he or she can consume no more than 500 calories worth of food and drink during these fasting days so that the body can maintain energy flow amongst other benefits.

If the individual engages in exercise, those days they workout should be reserved for the 5 or 6 free-eating days. The same goes for the 5:2 method. Try not to exercise (at least not excessively) on those days that are chosen for fasting. Your body will not appreciate the added stress when you're taking in so few calories. As always, you can choose to move up from eat-stop-eat to another method if this works easily and you're interested in something more advanced. Furthermore, you can start with a strict 24-hour method and then move up to a more flexible eat-stop-eat approach! Do what feels right, and never be afraid to troubleshoot one method for the sake of choosing another.

Alternate-Day Method

The alternate-day method is similar to the eat-stop-eat and 5:2 methods because it focuses on individual days "on" and "off" for fasting and eating. The difference for this method, in particular, is that it ends up being at least 2 days a week fasting, and sometimes, it can be as many as 4.

Some people follow very strict approaches to alternate-day method and literally fast every other day, only consuming 500 calories or less on those days designated for fasting. Some people, on the other hand, are much more flexible, and they tend to go for two days eating, one day fasting, two days eating, one day fasting, etc. The alternate-day method is even more flexible than the eat-stop-eat method in that sense, for it allows the individual to choose how he or she alternates between eating and fasting, based on what works for their body and mind the best.

The alternate-day method is like a step up from the eat-stop-eat and 24-hour methods, especially if the individual truly alternates between one-day fasting and the next day eating, etc. This more intense style of fasting works particularly well for people who are working on equally intense fitness regimens, surprisingly. People who are eating more calories a day than 2000 (which is true for a lot of bodybuilders and fitness buffs) will have more to gain from the alternate-day method, for you only have to cut back your eating on fasting days to about 25% of your standard caloric intake. Therefore, those fasting days can still provide solid nutritional support for fitness experts while helping them sculpt their bodies and maintain a new level of health.

Spontaneous Skipping Method

The alternate-day and eat-stop-eat methods are certainly flexible in their approaches to when the individual fasts and when he or she eats. However, none of those plans mentioned above are quite as flexible as the spontaneous skipping method. The spontaneous skipping method literally only requires that the individual skip meals within each day, whenever desired (and when it's sensed that the body can handle it).

Many people with more sensitive digestive systems or who practice more intense fitness regimens will start their experiences with IF through the spontaneous skipping method before moving on to something more intensive. People who have very haphazard daily schedules, or people who are around food a lot but forget to eat, will benefit from this method, for it works well with chaotic schedules and unplanned energies.

Despite that chaotic and unorganized potential, the spontaneous skipping method can also be more structured and organized, depending on what you make of it! For instance, someone desiring more structure can choose which meal each day they'd like to skip. Let's say he chooses to skip breakfast each day. Then, his spontaneous skipping method will be structured around making sure to skip breakfast (a.k.a.—not to eat until at least 12 pm) daily. Whatever you need to do to make this method work, try it! This method is made for experimentation and adventurousness.

Crescendo Method

The final method worth mentioning is the crescendo method, which is very well-suited for female practitioners (since their anatomies can be so detrimentally sensitive to high-intensity fasts). Essentially, this approach is made for internal awareness, gentle introductions, and gradual additions, depending on what works and what doesn't. It's a very active, trial-and-error type of method.

Through the crescendo method, the individual starts by only fasting 2 or 3 days a week, and on those fast days, it won't be a very intense fast at all. In fact, it wouldn't even be so strict that the individual would have to consume no more than 500 calories, like with the 5:2, eat-stop-eat, and other methods. Instead, these "fasting" days would be trial periods for methods like 12:12, 14:10, 16:8, or 20:4. The remaining 4 or 5 days out of the week would be open eating-window periods, but again, the practitioner is encouraged to maintain a healthy diet throughout the week.

The crescendo method works extremely well for female practitioners because it enables them to see how methods like

14:10 or 12:12 will affect their bodies without tying them to the method hook, line, and sinker. It allows them to see what each method does to their hormone levels, their menstruation tendencies, and their mood swings. Therefore, the crescendo method encourages these people to be more in touch with their bodies before moving too quickly into something that could do serious anatomical and hormonal damage.

The crescendo method will work extremely well for overweight or diabetic practitioners, too, for it will allow them to have these same "trial period" moments with all the methods before choosing what feels and works best, based on each individual situation.

Making Your Choice

When you make your choice from the 10 different options listed above, there are several things you'll want to keep in mind. First and foremost, amongst those things will be the fact that you can always choose another method (or a more flexible one to start with) in case something doesn't work as you'd hoped.

Ultimately, you'll also want to keep the following points in mind as you go about selecting your method: body type & abilities, lifestyle, daily tendencies, work routine, friends & family, and dietary choices. For all these considerations, remember what feels best to you, and remember to keep your goals with IF in mind at all times! If you ever feel like you're sacrificing your sanity or bodily health to attain these goals, go back to that step of troubleshooting, for you should never need to sacrifice those things to achieve any type of goal. Keep your eye on the prize and remember to choose what feels right, and see what works from there.

Consider your body type and abilities. Think of how your body looks and feels and how much about it you'd like to change. Think about how you react to food and what it looks like when you're hungry. Think about those things you view as your "limits" and how comfortable you are with pushing. Are you a fitness freak or a couch potato? Are you huskier or slimmer? Does your body hold onto fat or build muscle quickly? Do you retain water weight or not? Do you work out? Do you require a lot of water when you do? Consider all these things about your body and more, then compare them to the methods listed above. Compare them, too, to your overall goals with intermittent fasting to make sure that you're choosing a method that will help you actualize those goals as you conceive them. If you're looking to lose weight quickly, try a method that works with days "on" and "off" between fasting and eating. If you're looking to build muscle, the lean-gains method is probably the choice for you! If you're looking to boost your brain and heart, start with the crescendo method and see where it takes you!

Consider your lifestyle. When do you normally wake up and how much sleep do you get on an average night? How hungry are you normally when you wake up? How fast is your metabolism and when do you notice its peak? How do you make your living? Do you spend a lot of time in the car or on your feet or in an office? Are you constantly around other people or are you often alone? When you choose your method for intermittent fasting, make sure to consider all these lifestyle points. Maybe you wouldn't want to choose a method that disallows you to eat when you normally need the most energy. Maybe you wouldn't want to choose a method that forces you to eat when you're supposed to be at work. Most of these methods have a degree of choice and flexibility, so when you do find one you like, remember that you don't have to put yourself in a position that go against your nature (or circadian rhythms) to achieve any of your goals. Stay flexible, keep your goals in mind, and respect the norms of your body!

Consider your daily tendencies. Do you eat mostly in the daylight hours or after the sun goes down? Do you go to work in the daytime or nighttime? Are you generally nocturnal, diurnal, or crepuscular? Do you have a lot of freedom and flexibility in your daily routines? Do you travel a lot for work?

Do you spend a lot of time on the move? Do you have trouble remembering to eat? Are you the type of person that works out on the regular? Consider these themes in your life and more before you choose your method. Does it make sense for you to have low intake days where you consume 500 calories or less? Or does it make more sense for you to have extended periods in each day where you're not eating based on your habits or tendencies or otherwise? Plan something that makes sense and respects your habits so that the transition into intermittent fasting is as easy and painless as possible.

Consider your work routine. Do you go to work in the morning or night? Are you allowed to eat at work? Do you work around food or in the foodservice industry? Do you work on your feet all day or by doing something strenuous? Do you receive purposeful or accidental exercise opportunities at work or are you sitting in the same position all day? All these elements of your work routine will be important to consider as you decide which avenue of intermittent fasting to go down. You won't want to engage in a method like 20:4 if you're at work every day for incredibly short shifts. 20:4 works better for someone who works very long and distracting days. You won't want to try a method like 12:12 if part of your eating window involves being at work, when you're not allowed to eat at work. Remember to take your work life, routines, and restrictions into account when you go about making this choice. You will make things much less harsh on yourself if you can look at this bigger picture from the beginning and planning stages.

Consider your friends, coworkers, and family. How loud are their opinions? Are their lives oriented toward health? Do they demean you a lot or make fun of your choices? Or are they encouraging all of the time? Are these people your support system or are they your devils' advocates? Do you have the sense that they want to see you succeed? On the most basic level, are they nice to you and respectful of your choices? It might not seem that important, but the attitudes and supportive capacity of your friends, coworkers, and family can mean the world when you make a big choice like starting intermittent fasting. Sometimes, people just don't want to see us succeed. They block our successes with jealousy, pride, ignorance, or arrogance. When friends and family act like this, it's better to choose a method that allows you to avoid discussing IF around them whatsoever. When friends and family are open and supportive, they shouldn't influence your choice hardly at all. It's just when things are tenuous that you'll need to keep them (and your time around them) in consideration.

Finally, consider your dietary choices. Do you eat a lot of processed foods? Or do you eat a largely whole-foods, plant-based diet? Do you count calories? Do you cautiously skim nutrition facts? Are you looking for something specific like high fat, high fiber, or high protein? Are you hoping to change your diet entirely, or are you trying to keep things the way they are? Are you willing to sacrifice items of your diet to actualize your goals? All these questions help determine which type of method you're going to be ready for. If you're trying to change your diet entirely, a method with days "on" and days "off" will work best for you. In this case, try the 5:2, alternate-day, eat-stop-eat, or spontaneous skip methods. However, if you don't want to change your diet that much, a method where you fast for periods within each day will be desirable instead. Try methods like 20:4, 16:8, 14:10, or 12:12 for this type of situation.

As long as you make your selection with these 6 points in mind, you're sure to succeed with your intermittent fasting goals. You will enable yourself to make the safest, smartest, best choice for your circumstances, and that's an incredible tool to use in so many different applications. In this case, it's a tool that will help keep you healthy, boost your brain, heal your heart, and shed that excess weight like melted butter!

As a reminder, your first choice still might not be the right one. But, by making the most educated choice possible, you're sure to start from a good place and learn a lot about yourself regardless. Make sure you have a runner-up method (or two!) that's easy to swap to just in case the first one doesn't seem to show progress. Work smarter, not harder! Plan ahead, do the research, and know yourself. These are the truest steps to success that I know. And as always, don't be afraid to check with your doctor or nutritionist once the choice has been made. They'll be able to give you the final affirmation you need so you can get started on your new, healthy lifestyle with intermittent fasting in no time!

Autophagy

What Is Autophagy?

Autophagy is a process that happens within the human body that has been going on without our knowledge since the beginning of humanity. It is only recently that people have begun to harness this process in order to achieve desired and positive results through changes in their diet, such as intermittent fasting. We will look at this topic in-depth throughout this book, but here we will begin by looking at what exactly Autophagy is.

Autophagy, as a word, can be broken up into two individual parts. Each of these parts on its own is a separate Greek word—the word *auto*, which means self,and the word *phagy*, which means **the practice of eating.** Putting these together gives you **the practice of self-eating,** which is essentially what autophagy is. Now, this may sound a little intimidating, but it is a very natural process that our cells practice all the time without us being any the wiser. Autophagy is the body's way of cleaning itself out.

Essentially, the body has housekeepers that keep everything neat and tidy. Scientists who have been studying this for some time are now beginning to understand that there are ways to manipulate this process within your body in order to achieve things such as weight loss, improved health, reduction of disease symptoms, and so on. This is what we will spend the rest of the book looking at, but first, we will dive into the science of Autophagy a little more.

How Does Autophagy Work?

The process of autophagy involves small "hunter" particles that go around your body, looking for cells or cell components that are old and damaged. The hunter particles then take these cell components apart, getting rid of the damaged parts and saving the useful parts to make new cells later. These hunter cells can also use useful leftover parts to create energy for the body.

Autophagy has been found to happen in all organisms that are multi-cellular, like animals and plants, in addition to humans. While the study of these larger organisms and how autophagy works in their cells is lesser-known, more studies are being done on humans and how changes in diet can affect their body's autophagy.

The other function that autophagy serves is that it helps cells to carry out their death when it is time for them to die. There are times when cells are programmed to die because of a number of different factors. Sometimes these cells need assistance in their death, and autophagy can help them with this or can help to clean up after their death. The human body is all about life and death, and these processes are continually going on without our knowledge to keep us healthy and in good form.

The process of autophagy has been going on inside of us since our creation. This process has been kept around inside of our bodies because of the multitude of benefits it can provide us with. It is also essential for the health of our bodies, as being able to get rid of waste and damaged parts that are no longer useful to us is essential to our health. If we were unable to get rid of damaged or broken cells, these damaged particles would build up and eventually make us sick. Our bodies are extremely efficient in everything that they do, and waste disposal is no different.

More about autophagy and its relation to energy production has been studied in recent years, as this topic is of interest to humans. Autophagy can use old cell parts and recycle them to create new energy that the organism (like the human or animal) can then use to do its regular functions like walking and breathing. Now, people are studying what happens when humans rely on this form of energy production instead of the energy they would get from ingesting food throughout the day. This is where autophagy and intermittent fasting come together. We will look at how they work together throughout the rest of this book as we delve deeply into intermittent fasting and autophagy and how they work together to allow for things like weight loss or disease prevention.

What Does Autophagy Do?

Autophagy has many functions in the body. In this section, we will look at some of the other functions of autophagy and the body systems involved.

Autophagy is said to be the housekeeping function of the body. If you think of your body as your home, autophagy is the housekeeper that you hire to take care of all of the waste and the recycling functions of your cells.

One of the housekeeping duties includes removing cell parts that were built wrongly or at the wrong time. Sometimes cells make mistakes, and these mistakes can cause proteins or other cell parts to be formed in error. When this happens, we need something within the cell to get rid of these so that they do not take up space or get in the way of other processes within the cell. Furthermore, sometimes useful parts of the cell will become damaged and then will need to be removed in order to make way for a new part to take its place. These cell parts can include those that create DNA or those that create the proteins needed to make the DNA.

Another duty of autophagy is to protect the body from disease and pathogens. Pathogens are bacteria or viruses that can infect our cells and our bodies if they are not properly defended against. Autophagy works to kill the cells within our body that are infected by these pathogens in order to get rid of them before they can spread. In this way, autophagy plays a part in our immune system as it acts as a supplement to our immune cells whose sole function is to protect us from invasions by disease and infection.

Autophagy also functions to help the cells of the body to regulate themselves when there are stressors placed upon them. These stressors can be things like a lack of food for the cell or physical stresses placed on the cell. This regulation helps to maintain a standard cell environment despite factors that can change, like the availability of food. Autophagy is able to do things like break down cell parts for food to provide the cell with nutrients.

Similar to its role in the regulation of the cells, autophagy also helps with the development of a growing fetus inside of a woman's uterus. Autophagy occurs here to ensure that the embryo has enough nutrients and energy at all times for healthy development. In addition to this, it helps with growth in adults as well as there is a balance of building new parts and breaking down old ones involved in the growth of any organism.

Autophagy is more important than we may even realize, as it plays a large role in the survival of the living organisms it acts within. It does this by being especially sensitive to the levels of nutrients and energy within a cell. When the nutrient levels lower, autophagy breaks down cell parts, which creates nutrients and energy for the cell. If it weren't for this process, the cells would not be able to maintain their ideal functioning environment, and they may begin to make more mistakes and even lower their functioning abilities altogether. So much goes on inside of a cell that they need to be able to work effectively at all times. Autophagy makes this possible, which is what makes it such an essential function.

Using Intermittent Fasting to Induce Autophagy

Autophagy functions in the following way. When a decrease in nutrients is noticed within a cell, this decrease in nutrients acts as a signal for the cell to create small pockets within a membrane (a thin barrier layer) that are called **autophagosome**s. These small pockets (autophagosomes) move throughout the cell and find debris and damaged particles floating around within the cell. The small pockets then consume this debris by absorbing it into its inner space. The debris is then enclosed in the membrane (the thin barrier layer) and is moved to a place in the cell called the lysosome. A lysosome is a part of a cell that acts as a center for degradation, breakdown, or disassembly. This part of the cell gets debris and damaged cell parts delivered to it by the autophagosomes. Once these damaged cell parts are delivered, the lysosomes then break them down. By breaking them down, these parts can be recycled and used for energy.

The most common way to induce autophagy in a person is by way of starvation. This is not to say that a person must starve themselves, but that they starve their cells of nutrition temporarily. This is why people turn to fasting in order to induce autophagy. Low nutrition levels within the cells is the most common way that autophagy is triggered, as it is a process that creates energy within the cell. By knowing this, scientists have concluded that by inducing starvation within the cells, one can intentionally upregulate autophagy in their body. Intermittent fasting involves periods of fasting, which then induces a state of starvation within the cells (simply meaning that there is no energy being consumed to use for energy) and therefore induces autophagy in the cells to make energy.

Other Ways to Induce Autophagy

Starvation

The most common way to induce autophagy in a person is by way of starvation. Autophagy is triggered by a decrease in nutrients within a cell. As I mentioned above, the decrease in nutrients acts as a signal within the cell to begin the process of autophagy. This is exactly how intermittent fasting works.

Aerobic Exercise

One other way to activate autophagy is through exercise. Aerobic exercise has been shown through studies to increase autophagy in the cells of the muscles, heart, brain, lungs, and the liver.

Sleep

Sleep is very important for autophagy. If you have ever gone a few days without a proper, restful sleep, you know that you begin to feel a decline in your mental abilities quickly. This could be because of your brain's decreased autophagy functioning. The number of hours that you are in bed does not matter if the sleep is not good quality, though. Quality sleep for the right number of hours is what is needed to maintain good brain function and keep your brain's autophagy going.

Specific Foods

The consumption of specific foods has been shown to induce or promote autophagy. The added benefit is that not only do they trigger autophagy in the cells of your body, these foods are also shown to have numerous other health benefits.

Exercising for Women over 50

Many people will ask if it is safe to combine fasting with exercise. I am here to say it is. However, some factors need to be considered before combining the two. First, the type of fasting regimen should be considered alongside the physical, mental, and psychological health of the individual. Women with existing medical conditions should not combine fasting with exercise before being advised by a medical expert. So, while it is safe to practice intermittent fasting and include exercise, if you are an already active person, doing so is not suitable for everyone.

Firstly, your metabolism can be negatively impacted if you exercise and fast for long periods of time. For example, if you exercise daily while fasting for more than a month, your metabolic rate can begin to slow down. So, while it may sound like a quick way to reap the benefits of your limited calorie intake, moderation is crucial.

Combining the two can trigger a higher rate of breaking down glycogen and body fat. This means that you burn fat at an accelerated rate. Also, when you combine these two, your growth hormones are boosted. This results in improved bone density. Your muscles are also positively impacted when you exercise. Your muscles will become more resilient to stress and age slower. This is also a quick way to trigger autophagy keeping brain cells and tissues strong, making you feel, and look younger.

Cardiovascular exercise is great for the heart and lungs. It improves oxygen delivery to specific parts of your body, reduces stress, improves sleep, burns fat, and improves sex drive. Among the more common cardio exercises are brisk walking, running, and swimming. In the gym, machines such as the elliptical, treadmill, and StairMaster are used to help with cardio. Some people are satisfied and feel like they've done enough after 20 minutes on the treadmill. However, if you want to continue to be strong and independent as you grow older, you need to consider adding strength training to your workout. After 50, strength training for a woman is no longer about six-pack abs, building biceps, or vanity muscles. Instead, it has switched to maintaining a body that is healthy, strong, and is less prone to injury and illnesses.

Strength Training Exercises for Women Over 50

These ten strength training exercises listed below are ones you can do right in the comfort of your own home. All you need is a mat, a chair, and some hand weights of about 3 – 8 pounds. As you get stronger, you can increase the weight. Take a minute to rest before switching between each routine. Ensure that you move slowly through the exercises, breathe properly, and focus on maintaining the right form. If you start to feel lightheaded or dizzy during your routines, especially if you are performing the exercise during your fasting window, discontinue immediately.

Squat to Chair

This exercise is great for improving your bone health. A lot of age-related bone fractures and falls in women involve the pelvis, so this exercise will target and strengthen your pelvic bone and the surrounding muscles.

To perform this:

1. Stand fully upright in front of a chair as if you are ready to sit and spread your feet shoulder-width apart.

2. Extend your arms in front of you and keep them that way all through the movement.

3. Bend your knees and slowly lower your hips as if you want to sit on the chair, but don't sit. When your butt

touches the chair slightly, press into your heels to get back your initial standing position. Repeat that for about 10 to 15 times.

Forearm Plank

This exercise targets your core and shoulders.

Here's how to do it:

1. Get into a push-up position, but with your arms bent at the elbows such that your forearm is supporting your weight.

2. Keep your body off the mat or floor and keep your back straight at all times. Don't raise or drop your hips. This will engage your core. Hold the position for 30 seconds and then drop to your knees. Repeat ten times.

Modified Push-ups

This routine targets your arms, shoulders, and core.

Here's how to do it:

1. Kneel on your mat. Place your hands on the mat below your shoulders and let your knees be behind your hips so that your back is stretched at an angle.

2. Tuck your toes under and tighten your abdominal muscles. Gradually bend your elbows as you lower your chest toward the floor.

3. Push back on your arms to press your chest back to your previous position. Repeat for as many times as is comfortable.

Bird Dog

When done correctly, this exercise can strengthen the muscles of your posterior chain as it targets your back and core. It may seem easy at first but can be a bit tricky.

To do this correctly:

1. Go on all fours on your mat.

2. Tighten your abdominal muscles and shift your weight to your right knee and left hand. Slowly extend your right hand in front of you and your left leg behind you. Ensure that both your hands and legs are extended as far as possible and stay in that position for about 5 seconds. Return to your starting position. This is one repetition. Switch to your left knee and right hand and repeat the movement. Alternate between both sides for 20 repetitions.

Shoulder Overhead Press

This targets your biceps, shoulders, and back.

To perform this move:

1. With dumbbells in both hands, stand and spread your feet shoulder-width apart.

2. Bring the dumbbells up to the sides of your head and tighten your abdominal muscles.

3. Slowly press the dumbbells up until your arms are straight above your head. Slowly return to the first position. Repeat 10 times. You can also do this exercise while sitting.

Chest Fly

This targets your chest, back, core, and glutes.

To do this:

1. Lie with your back flat on your mat, your knees at an angle close to 90 degrees, and your feet firmly planted on the floor or mat.

2. Hold dumbbells in both hands over your chest. Keep your palms facing each other and gently open your hands away from your chest. Let your upper arms touch the floor without releasing the tension in them.

3. Contract your chest muscles and slowly return the dumbbells to the initial position. Repeat about ten times.

Standing Calf Raise

This exercise improves the mobility of your lower legs and feet as well as improves your stability.

Here's how to perform it.

1. *Hold a dumbbell in your left hand and place your right hand on something sturdy to give you balance.*

2. *When you are sure of your balance, lift your left foot off the floor with the dumbbell hanging at your side. Stand erect and move your weight such that you are almost standing on your toes.*

3. Slowly return to the starting position. Do this 15 times before switching to the other leg and doing the same thing all over again.

Single-Leg Hamstring Bridge

This move targets your glutes, quads, and hamstrings.

To do this:

1. Lie flat on your back. Place your feet flat on mat or the floor and spread your bent knees apart.

2. Place your arms flat by your side and lift one leg straight.

3. Contract your glutes as you lift your hips into a bridge position with your arms still in position. Hold for about 2 to 3 seconds and drop your hips to the mat. Repeat about ten times before switching your leg. Do the same again.

Bent-Over Row

This targets your back muscles and spine.

To do this:

1. Hold dumbbells in both hands and stand behind a sturdy object (for example, a chair). Bend forward and rest your head on the chosen object. Relax your neck and slightly bend your knees. With both palms facing each other pull the dumbbells to touch your ribs. Hold the position for about 2 to 5 seconds and slowly return to the starting position. Repeat 10 to 15 times.

Basic Ab

A distended belly is a common occurrence in older women. This exercise can strengthen and tighten the abdominal muscles bringing them inward toward your spine.

To perform this:

2. Lie on your back with your feet firmly planted on the floor and your knees bent. Relax your upper body and rest your hands on your thighs.

3. As you exhale, lift yourself upward off the mat or floor. Stop the upward movement when your hands are resting on your knees. Hold the position for about 2 to 5 seconds and then slowly return to the starting position. Repeat for about 20 to 3o times.

Including Exercises in Your Daily Routine

You do not have to hit the gym or plan a time dedicated to working out. You can make exercise part of your daily routine so that you are always getting the proper amount of body movement, whether or not it is time for exercise.

Tips on how to include exercises into your daily routine.

- Take the stairs (within reason) instead of using the elevator. You don't want to go up a ten-story building using the stairs! If you have a long way to go up or down, take the stairs a couple of flights and then complete your trip with the elevator.

- When you talk with your family members at home, don't shout from the top floor and bottom floor. Go up or climb down and talk with them.

- Find a sporting activity that you thoroughly enjoy and do it as often as is convenient. When you're doing something you enjoy, you'll hardly think of it as exercise, and you're likely to stay committed.

- If you are at work, instead of sending emails or text messages to coworkers, walk up to them and talk to them face to face.

- If possible, convert your one-on-one meetings to a walking meeting. Hold the meeting while taking a stroll outside.

- Stop a block or two from your destination and walk the rest of the way. Make walking your preferred mode of transportation.

- Take your dog for walks daily. If you don't have a dog, adopt one. It might seem that you are merely walking your dog, but you are also exercising your muscles.

- Take brisk walks as often as possible. Remember to put on comfortable shoes when walking briskly. You can bring your walking shoes with you to make it easy for you to change into them.

Staying Safe While Combining Intermittent Fasting and Exercise

Exercising in your fasting window can help you quickly achieve some of the advanced benefits of intermittent fasting. Nevertheless, it is crucial to follow a few general guidelines to keep you safe during the practice.

There are no iron-cast rules about when to exercise even on fasting days. Observe what works well for you whether exercising before eating (during the fasting window) or eating before working out (during the eating window). Many women find that exercising on an empty stomach suits their body and leaves them feeling energized for the rest of the day. If this is your preferred method, set aside time in the morning before your first meal of the day. Some other women find that although they prefer working out on an empty stomach, they feel depleted right after the exercise. In that case, shift your exercise to about 20 to 30 minutes before your first meal of the day. Your body would have rested a bit after your exercise before you break your fast.

If you prefer working out after you break your fast that is perfectly fine. Eating shortly before your exercise doesn't render your exercises ineffective. Remember that all of our bodies work in different ways. Keep in mind that the goal of working out is to maintain proper body health long into your golden years. You don't need to impress anyone with great abs or biceps, instead impress yourself with how much power you have. Stay committed to your routines, but don't overdo it. If you start feeling weak, that is your cue to take a break.

If you are fasting for longer periods (24 hours or more), you will need to conserve your energy. Consider doing exercises that will not exert too much stress. For example, take a walk, do some yoga, or any other type of low-intensity exercise.

We could all use someone on our shoulder reminding us to drink more water. And going without food reduces your body's water content even more. Add in higher levels of exertion and you'll be depleting your water reserves very quickly. So here is your reminder to always drink adequate amounts of water before, during, and after your workout sessions.

Intermittent Fasting and Hormones

For women over 50, there are several hormones that come into play by this age. Some of these hormones are reduced while we age, while others are overly active. Intermittent fasting can help you regulate each of these hormones to their optimum. Let's see how each hormone gets affected or reacts through intermittent fasting techniques.

Food and Appetite Hormones

We have seen the effects of intermittent fasting on insulin and how it helps counter insulin resistance. Let's now see how intermittent fasting can help another resistance phenomenon known as Leptin Resistance. Leptin, as we know is the satiety hormone, tells us when we have had enough food and need to stop. However, due to various eating disorders and hormonal changes in our body, our brain stops listening to leptin telling us to stop. Though leptin is secreted at normal levels and is actively present in the bloodstream, our body fails to recognize that it is full and there is no further need for food.

This disorder leads to more and more consumption of food and naturally leads to abnormal weight gains. Intermittent fasting can help you counter leptin resistance. When you are fasting regularly, you are gaining a sense of self-control and denying the twisted signals of the hunger hormone. Through continued intermittent fasting you will be able to pass up a plate of cake or your favorite chocolate ice cream without falling into the urge of taking a bite. Because your brain was refusing to listen to normal levels of leptin, your body was producing it in high amounts which still went ignored. But through intermittent fasting, you will be able to scale down your leptin levels making you highly sensitive to even small levels of this hormone. This is what will make you feel full when you have had a good meal. Eating more fiber-rich foods, and low-carb diets can be crucial in this scenario.

The hunger hormone, ghrelin also undergoes considerable changes during fasts. These changes have been known to have positive effects on dopamine levels which in turn improve concentration and cognitive abilities.

Female Reproductive Hormones

Estrogen and Progesterone are the female hormones responsible for various reproductive functions. For women who are younger and still in the childbearing or menstruating age, intermittent fasting has varying effects. For some women, intermittent fasting has been known to be great and non-inhibitory in terms of their reproductive hormones. For other women, who were too sensitive to intermittent fasting, it can result in disturbed periods or temporary infertility. But, for women who are over the age of 50, this concern disappears as these women no longer produce much estrogen and are beyond the menstruating age. Therefore, period irregularity or infertility are no longer a concern.

A healthy brain-ovary axis is what determines the health of a woman with respect to the female hormones. For women over 50, without the concerns of disturbing these hormones, intermittent fasting helps maintain a healthy brain-ovary axis to ensure good hormone health.

Even for those who have not yet crossed menopause, intermittent fasting is not risky. It all comes down to how you introduce intermittent fasting to your body. Taking things slowly is essential. As your body gets accustomed to smaller fasting periods you can gradually move to longer fasts. It has been shown through research that all hormonal irregularity occur when you send your body into shock through fasting for longer periods suddenly. Give yourself, and your body, sufficient time to get acclimatized to the concept of fasting and you won't need to fear any hormonal imbalance due to your fasts.

Adrenal Hormones

Adrenal hormones are the hormones released by the adrenal glands. The adrenal glands are situated over the kidneys and are responsible for regulating our moods in times of stress, anxiety, and excitement. Of these hormones, the most important is the stress hormone, also known as cortisol. A healthy adrenal-brain axis, or the HPA axis, is necessary to have regulated levels of adrenal hormones. When this balance is disturbed, cortisol levels spike up irregularly or go too low. This is observed to happen with intermittent fasting for longer durations of time. Cortisol levels may swing dangerously to either extreme, increasing the stress levels in our body. This leads to a condition that is commonly known as adrenal fatigue. The most common symptoms of adrenal fatigue are tiredness, muscle weakness, extreme nervousness, sleep issues, and digestive problems.

The HPA axis disturbance can give rise to several circadian rhythm issues. People who are already suffering from circadian rhythm problems find intermittent fasting for prolonged periods highly stressful. For these people, it is highly recommended to follow the crescendo method of fasting. Taking it slowly and increasing your fasting hours gradually can be the key to having well-regulated cortisol levels so as to keep stress at bay.

Thyroid Hormones

The thyroid consists of two lobes on either side of the throat, connected by a small bridge-like tissue. When thyroid function is normal, it is nearly impossible to feel your thyroid by physical examination. In conditions such as hypothyroidism and Hashimoto's, which is an autoimmune thyroid issue, the thyroid is often easily felt.

Research has shown that intermittent fasting, that included fasting hours during the night and the eating window during the day, had positive improving effects on hypothyroid problems. The thyroid gland is controlled and regulated by the body's internal biological clock which is also known as the circadian rhythm. Keeping the circadian rhythm functioning normally is essential to having normal thyroid functions. Therefore, if the fast can be observed so as to not disturb the body's inherent biological clock, then it can work in the favor of those suffering from thyroid issues.

It was observed that when the fast was elongated beyond the 16-hour mark, the circadian rhythms were disturbed, and this affected the proper functioning of the thyroid gland in those suffering from hypothyroidism. Longer fasts of around 24 hours or more are highly inappropriate for patients with dysfunctional thyroid activity. Therefore, for hypothyroid patients, it is advisable that they fast only for 14 to 16 hours and make it a point to have their eating window during the day. This will help balance their thyroid functioning and regulate their already irregular thyroid hormone levels.

7 common errors to avoid

It is impossible to escape what seems to some to be a fashion effect. Everyone talks about intermittent fasting. I'm not going to make yet another copy of the hundreds of books already existing on the subject that only list the main benefits of intermittent fasting. If you have just come out of several years of hibernation and are still ignorant about it, a simple search on Google will fill all of your gaps.

In this book, I want to talk to you about three big mistakes that seem to be recurring. This will perhaps prevent you, too, from riding the wave of "fasting"... and burning fat without needing to snack throughout the 2 hours. Intermittent fasting is an art.

Mistake #1: Abusing Stimulants (Coffee, Tea, Etc.)

In the world of intermittent fasting, it is generally accepted that you can eat or drink whatever you want as long as the food or drink contains no calories. Indeed, the goal of the fasting phase is to keep your insulin low to maintain the fat-burning mode. We know that lipids stimulate **a little**, proteins **moderately**, and carbohydrates a **lot** of insulin.

Remember: when the **insulin is high**, your body is in **storage** mode; when **insulin is low**, your body is in a **destocking** mode (fat burning).

If we stop there, any drink containing no calories is eligible for the fasting phase: tea, coffee, drinks containing false sugars. Stimulating drinks are also often recommended by several promoters of intermittent fasting. Caffeine is indeed well known in the world of fitness and food supplements to suppress appetite and speed up metabolism. In theory, it also has a potential bonus in terms of fat loss.

I have absolutely nothing against coffee lovers, having myself been a chronic drinker a few years ago. Still, we know very well that as a psychotropic drug, caffeine is nothing but legal doping. The fact that its consumption is culturally accepted does not change the fact that it is antinomy to fasting (intermittent or not) in terms of health.

The Harmful Effects of Caffeine in the Long Term

To understand the harmful effects, let's already briefly summarize the action of caffeine on the body. Caffeine will take the place of a neuromodulator, adenosine, which usually has the role of slowing down nervous activity if necessary (energy deficit) while stimulating the action of the adrenal glands (production of adrenaline). In other words, coffee, and tea to a lesser extent, will produce a peak of energy by preventing the signal of fatigue from playing its role. A message, which is not there to annoy us but rather to protect our potentially significant damage to the body, which could occur as a result of over-activity in the nervous system.

Coffee is a popular but not harmless drink for our health.

Concretely, when a person's nervous system begins to exhaust itself for various reasons (chronic lack of sleep or overwork, for example), the short-term "beneficial" effects of caffeine will become more and more felt. The person then becomes addicted to their little daily boost of caffeine and may start to multiply the cups during the day. After a few years of overwork, the person is so exhausted that they begin to manifest symptoms of caffeine intolerance more and more marked:

- Tachycardia

- Nervousness

- Mood swings

- Intestinal disorders

- Cravings

If you are in the latter case, the consumption of caffeine will cause stress such that your hormonal system will cause an increase in blood sugar (and therefore insulin), by going to draw on your lean mass. You will consequently, potentially, lose muscle and cravings while stopping to draw on your body fat. Everything you want to avoid when you fast to improve your body composition!

I'm Drinking Coffee! Is It a Severe, Doctor?

Firstly, I am not a doctor. But my point of view is that we do not live in a perfect world. So if you choose to consume stimulants, do so knowing it is as if you take out an (energy) loan. When you borrow from your bank, the money you borrow will have to be paid back at some point. If you combine credits on credits, you know that you will end up having big problems. The same will apply if you take stimulants on a daily and exaggerated basis.

Sweeteners Drinks: The False Good Idea

A word on drinks containing false sugars. We have known for a few years now that despite the absence of calories, sweeteners lure the body by stimulating the production of insulin. Their consumption, therefore, indirectly promotes insulin resistance. Fasting, on the contrary, promotes its recovery. We are not even talking here about the neurotoxic effect of these substances, which is no longer to be proven. These drinks are, therefore, entirely counterproductive in the context of intermittent fasting.

If you suspect chronic fatigue at home and wish to experience intermittent fasting, avoid trying to cheat by using stimulants, especially on an empty stomach. This will only slow down your results by worsening your fatigue. Once weaned from caffeine, and your nervous system rested, you will have equally vital energy (if not more) on an empty stomach, and above all, much more stable over time!

Do you need to wake up your metabolism in the morning? Move, breathe, walk, run, and swim! Natural stimulations will produce more beneficial and lasting results over time than purely chemical and addictive stimulation of caffeine. Currently, in the summer, I like the contact with cold water every morning. This puts me in good condition for the rest of the day. It's up to you to find what suits you!

Mistake #2: Wanting to Do Too Much

Many people go headlong into the single meal mode because they have been told that it is the best of the best. That they will live ten times longer and lose a hundred times more fat. As often, the excess of enthusiasm hides a more nuanced reality.

In reality, you will only get results that match what your body can currently support, depending on your level of vitality. There is only one rule: you must feel good. If you are calm and concentrated at the same time, and you do not feel hunger at all, these are signs that your body is drawing in its fats. You can continue to fast and do it naturally because it is easy for you.

But, if on the other hand, you start to become stressed for no apparent reason, have difficulty concentrating, become irritable, have obsessive thoughts for food, this is undoubtedly the sign that you have exceeded your capacity for adaptation (to the lack of glucose). Your cortisol levels get carried away, and your stress level can potentially become destructive. You can also recognize yourself in this description if, when you are refueling, you experience hyperplasic disorders. The problem is not intermittent fasting, but the fact that you have set the bar too high.

Being too rigid on schedules can be counterproductive.

I noticed how my ability to fast was reduced to nothing if, for one reason or another, I went through a period of fatigue or lack of sleep. In this case, I do not feel guilty, and I eat to get fuel and do my daily activities. Conversely, when I am well-rested, I can sometimes eat nothing until the evening without even thinking about it. Intermittent fasting is a great tool, but it is not magical and should not become a religion. You do not have to practice it strictly 365 days a year to get the benefits.

Note that I am not speaking here of therapeutic fasting in the classical sense of the term. The purposes are not precisely the same. In intermittent, daily fasting, we aim to optimize metabolism above all and wish to remain active.

And What about the Warrior Diet?

You can consume during the day a small portion of foods with a low glycemic index (example: a handful of berries, a glass of vegetable juice), as well as meals with little digestive impact, in small quantities. This approach is notably recommended by Ori Hofmekler, author of the "Warrior Diet", and one of the people known to have significantly contributed to popularizing intermittent fasting in our modern era.

If you choose to test the Warrior Diet, don't forget the keyword: **control**. The risk in adopting this strategy is to generate cravings for compulsive snacking and to cancel the benefits of the period of restriction. Indeed, even fruits and vegetable juices can cause a significant rise in blood sugar, and therefore, insulin is not a problem in absolute terms. Still, when you fast, you want to keep your insulin as low as possible to prevent burning your fat stores.

So, is the "Warrior Diet" for you? If you can control yourself and settle for a handful of berries without waking you up for the rest of the day, why not? Otherwise, in my experience, it is better to reserve fruits and vegetables for during the feeding window.

If you exceed your adaptability by wanting to push the fast too far in the day, you risk obtaining the opposite effects of those sought. Go gradually, like starting out by skipping breakfast. For example, the body needs time to learn how to use its fat stores. Wanting to go too fast means taking the risk of spending your days without the energy to depress and ultimately give up. Play and progress with intermittent fasting without making it a dogma.

Mistake #3: Not Eating Enough after Breaking the Fast

As much as you must be on a food restriction during the fasting phase, as much as during the compensation phase, you must eat enough, whether in one or more doses. Do not be afraid of eating enough in the evening, thinking that you are going to store fat. It is a legend linked to the fact that most people snack all day long. Limiting yourself in the evening in the latter context will have a beneficial impact. But, when we fast a significant part of the day, we are in a completely different meaning.

Be careful, it is, of course, not a question of gorging yourself and gobbling up everything that comes your way, especially just before sleeping, at the risk of spending your night (poorly) digesting. Eating in serenity with proper chewing is always a must. If you cannot control yourself, I refer you to the previous point.

Intermittent fasting also does not slow down the metabolism in the long term as we sometimes hear it in the mouths of its detractors. Once again, if we eat enough during the compensation phase.

Do not make restrictions during the compensation phase.

How Do I Know If I'm Eating Enough with One or Two Meals a Day?

If you are doing the "single meal" mode (4 to 6-hour food window, for example), think about large family meals or when you go to a restaurant. Take your time! A "single meal" does not necessarily mean a single plate or a single food intake. A little tip from Ori: allow at least 20 to 30 minutes (or more) to pass after each food intake. This is the time generally necessary for the signal of satiety to rise to the brain. If hunger returns after this time, you can continue eating. However, avoid eating all of your calories just before sleeping for reasons that you will quickly understand (digestion).

One of the main benefits of intermittent fasting is that it allows you to reconnect with your real hunger. Learn to listen to it without locking yourself into overly complicated protocols that don't suit your needs. The quality of your **digestion**, your **sleep,** as well as your **energy** and your daily **mood** being four good indicators allowing you to know if you are doing things the right way or not.

Mistake #4: Being Impatient

Whatever propaganda you may have heard about fast results, the reality is that nothing is typical because we all have unique processes regardless of our physical appearance. Be patient, even if others who began fasting at the same time as you are already seeing results and you have nothing to show for your efforts so far. It can be frustrating and discouraging but give your body time to adjust. As long as you don't have any medical reason to stop, don't give up. Continue the practice for at least a month.

Realize that changes take time. There is no magic about the process of losing weight, improved vitality, or any other health benefits of intermittent fasting. Don't be in a hurry, and don't give people the room to put you under unnecessary pressure. Each person has their own pace, and it has absolutely nothing to do with you. If you continue to focus on other people's results, or your seeming lack of results, you are giving your mind reasons to discontinue. Be patient.

Mistake #5: Fussing Over What You Can Eat

One common mistake people make when fasting is obsessing over the fasting hours and what to eat when they are finally allowed. You don't have to worry about if you are fasting as long as someone else, the important thing is what's comfortable for you. Of course, if your fasting window is too small, you are not likely to see any result. Also, don't get too tied up in every little detail of intermittent fasting. For example, you don't have to become too worried because you missed a day. Remember that fasting intermittently should be a lifestyle change if you want to continue to reap the benefits. And for a lifestyle change to be sustainable, you must be able to adapt and use it in a way that even if you face challenges, you will work your way around it somehow. Missing a day or cutting your fast short for reasons beyond your control shouldn't get you worked up and worrying about whether you can do the entire plan. Don't give up.

Again, some people focus too much on what they can or cannot eat. For example, "Can I add just a little butter or cream?" "Would it hurt to eat this type of food during the fasting window?" If your focus is on what you can have or eat while you are fasting, you are giving your attention to the wrong things and putting your mind in an unhelpful state. Give your mind the right focus by concentrating on doing a good, clean, fast, and try to consume only water, tea, or coffee during the fasting window.

Mistake #6: Not Monitoring Your Hormones

A woman's hormones can be easily thrown out of whack by the slightest change in her already established pattern of behavior. Whether it is a physical change, such as altering you're eating pattern, or an emotional change, such as being irritated or sad, it can bring about hormonal imbalance in a woman even if it is temporary.

For premenopausal and menopausal women, hormones can go haywire for reasons even they cannot define. She could be feeling great all week, and without anything changing she could suddenly become fatigued, depressed, and not in the right frame of mind. These changes happen due to the unpredictability of this phase of a woman's life. Because this can happen for no apparent reason, it is best to check your hormonal levels before putting your body through a major lifestyle change. If you've ever had issues with thyroid, cortisol, or adrenal fatigue, ensure that you have these checks before you begin intermittent fasting.

This could be a surprise to some women, but your ovaries produce testosterone too. So, as you grow older and begin to experience a decline in your estrogen and progesterone levels, your testosterone levels are also taking a nosedive. Your libido can be affected by low levels of testosterone and make you feel exhausted and bummed-out for no reason at all. So, while you are checking your other hormones, don't forget to do a testosterone test as well. The thyroid and testosterone hormones can also help in weight regulation. So, if you intend to shed some weight using intermittent fasting, these tests are necessary.

Mistake #7: Not Starting Slow

To go from having five or six meals daily to eating only once a day can lead to very dire consequences. Apart from being harmful to your health, massive abrupt changes are hardly sustainable. After confirming that intermittent fasting is suitable for your health, the next thing to do is to plan how to ease into the habit. Take another look at the example of how to ease into fasting in Chapter 2 and consider following the example or coming up with something similar that works for you. In other words, before you fully implement any intermittent fasting regimen, it is a good practice to first test the waters, so to speak, with a less strict form of fasting. By doing this, it will help your body acclimate to the changes before going into the proper regimen.

Precautions to Take while on IF

Find a Worthy Goal

First things first: find a goal that is worth pursuing, or else you will drop the idea at the first sign of resistance. If you don't have a goal that represents a strong ideal, it won't be long before you start telling yourself, "I think I've passed the stage of such childishness." Many women start a new lifestyle change for reasons that they can't keep up with when things get tough. For example, the desire to look like models on TV, or social media makes losing weight feel socially acceptable and ok to keep up with trends that can be harmful. These reasons are not enough to keep anyone committed to a full lifestyle change and few wonder why so many people with goals are quick to jump from one lifestyle to another.

Don't go into fasting intermittently because it is the thing to do at the moment. Instead, look for inspiring goals such as:

- Staying fit, young, and healthy.

- Improving your cognitive or brain functions.

- Improving your overall vitality and increase energy levels.

- Balancing hormones, especially during menopausal or post-menopausal stages of life.

- Improving your overall health, thereby increasing longevity.

Do any of these sounds good to you? Surely at this stage of your life, you are aware of the inherent risks of doing something merely because others are doing it too. That type of motivation will fail you.

Watch Electrolytes

Body electrolytes are compounds and elements that occur naturally in body fluids, blood, and urine. They can also be ingested through drinks, foods, and supplements. Some of them include magnesium, calcium, potassium, chloride, phosphate, and sodium. Their functions include fluid balance, regulation of the heart and neurological function, acid-base balance, oxygen delivery, and many other functions.

It is important to keep these electrolytes in a state of balance. But many people who practice fasting tend to neglect this and run into problems. Here is a common notion: "Don't let anything into your stomach until the end of your fast." Even those just starting to fast know it doesn't work that way, and they tend to forget or fully stay away from liquids during their fasting window.

When you lose too much water from your body through sweating, vomiting, and diarrhea, or you don't have enough water in your body because you don't drink enough liquids, you increase the risk of electrolyte disorders. It is not okay to drink tea or black coffee throughout the morning period of your fast window. You will wear down if you do not drink enough water. The longer you fast without water, the higher your chances of flushing out electrolytes and running into trouble. You can end up raising your blood pressure, develop muscle twitching and spasms, fatigue, fast heart rate or irregular heartbeat, and many other health problems.

In contrast, drinking too much water can also tip the water-electrolyte balance. What you want to do is to drink adequate amounts of water and not drink an excess water, whether you are fasting or not.

Give the Calorie Restriction a Rest

Remember that intermittent fasting is different from dieting. Your focus should be on eating healthily during your eating window or eating days instead of focusing on calorie restriction. Even if you are fasting for weight loss, don't obsess over calories. Following a fasting regimen is enough to take care of the calories you consume. It is unnecessary to engage in a practice that can hurt your metabolism. Combining intermittent fasting with eating too little food in your eating window because you are worried about your calorie intake can cause problems for your metabolism.

One of the major reasons that people push themselves into restricting calories while fasting is their concern for rapid weight loss. You need to be wary of any process that brings about drastic physical changes to your body in very short amounts of time. While it is okay to desire quick results, your health and safety are more important. When you obsess or worry that you are not losing weight as quickly as you want, you are not helping matters. Instead, you are increasing your stress level which becomes counterproductive. You are already taking practical steps toward losing weight by intermittent fasting, why would you want to undo your hard work by unnecessary worrying?

Simply focus on following a sustainable intermittent fasting regimen and let go of the need to restrict your calorie intake. Intermittent fasting will give your body the right number of calories it needs if you do it properly.

The First Meal of the Eating Window is Key

Breaking your fast is a crucial part of the process because if you don't get it right, it could quickly develop into unhealthy eating patterns. When you break your fast, it is important to have healthy foods around to prevent yourself from grabbing unhealthy feel-good snacks. Make sure what you are eating in your window is not a high-sugar or high-carb meal. I recommend that you consider breaking your fast with something that is highly nutrient-dense such as a green smoothie, protein shake, or a healthy salad.

As much as possible, avoid breaking your fast with foods from a fast-food restaurant. Eating junk foods after your fast is a quick way to ruin all the hard work you've put in during your fasting window. If, for any reason, you can't prepare your meal, ensure that you order very specific foods that will complement your effort and not destroy what you've built.

Break Your Fast Gently

It is okay to feel very hungry after going for a long time without food, even if you were drinking water all through the fasting window. This is particularly true for people who are just starting with fasting. But don't let the intensity of your hunger push you to eat. You don't want to quickly force food into your stomach after going long without food, or you might hurt yourself and experience stomach distress. Take it slow when you break your fast. Eat light meals in small portions when you first break your fast. Wait for a couple of minutes for your stomach to get used to the presence of food again before continuing with a normal-sized meal. The waiting period will douse any hunger pangs and remove the urge to rush your meal. For example, break your fast with a small serving of salad and wait for about fifteen minutes. Drink some water and then after about five more minutes, you can eat a normal-sized meal.

Nutrition is Important

Although intermittent fasting is not dieting and so, does not specify which foods to eat, limit, and completely avoid, it makes sense to eat healthily. This means focusing on eating a balanced diet, such as:

- Whole grains

- Fruits and vegetables (canned in water, fresh, or frozen).

- Lean sources of protein (lentils, beans, eggs, poultry, tofu, and so on).

- Healthy fats (nuts, seeds, coconuts, avocados, olive oil, olive, and fatty fish).

It simply doesn't make any sense to go for 16 hours (or more) without food and then spend the rest of the day eating junk. Even if you follow the 5:2 method and limit your calorie intake to only 500 calories per day for two days, it is totally illogical to follow it with five days of eating highly processed foods and low-quality meals. Combining intermittent fasting with unbalanced diets will lead to nutritional deficiencies and defeat the goal of fasting in the first place. Realize that intermittent fasting is not a magic wand that makes all poor eating habits vanish in a poof! For the practice to work, you must be deliberate about the types of food you eat.

Find a Regimen That Works for You

Don't follow a fasting plan because it seems to suit someone else. Instead, go for something that fits into your schedule. If you feel caged or boxed in by a particular fasting plan, it is a clear indication that it is not a suitable plan for you. Thankfully, you have the freedom to design something that can work for you, even if you are following a specific regimen. The regimens are not carved in stone! They are flexible, and you can adjust them to suit you as long as you follow each regimen's basic principles. For example, if you decide to follow the 16:8 fasting regimen, your 8-hour eating window does not need to be strictly between noon and 8 pm. You have the option of tailoring the eating window to something that gives you room to handle other aspects of your life, such as work, hobbies, family, and so on. You might decide to make your 8-hour eating window from 9 am to 5 pm, or from 1 pm to 9 pm.

Whatever you choose to do is totally up to you. After all, it is your life, and you have the freedom to choose what you want. Books, the internet, and even loved ones can only suggest and offer recommendations. Ultimately, the final decision rests with you. Since your goal is not to please someone else or seek external approval, you should make your choice based on what is most convenient for you. You are seeking results, not accolades. Therefore, don't follow something unrealistic for you or is too restrictive. Even if you endure the most stringent type of fast and get admiration and commendation from others, have you considered what that fasting regimen is doing to your overall health? The female body is delicately designed, and putting it through unnecessary stress is unsafe if you are merely enduring discomfort to boost your ego.

Myths About Intermittent Fasting

Skipping Breakfast Makes You Fat

One progressing fantasy is that the morning meal is the most significant meal of the day.

Individuals normally accept that skipping breakfast prompts unnecessary yearning, desires, and weight gain. One 16-week study in 283 grown-ups with overweight and heftiness watched no weight distinction between the individuals who had breakfast and the individuals who didn't. Consequently, breakfast doesn't generally influence your weight, despite the fact that there might be some individual changeability. A few examinations even recommend that individuals who get thinner over the long haul will, in general, have breakfast. Also, kids and young people who have breakfast will, in general, perform better at school. Thusly, it's imperative to focus on your specific needs. Breakfast is gainful for certain individuals, while others can skip it with no negative outcomes.

Eating Often Supports Your Digestion

Numerous individuals accept that eating more dinners builds your metabolic rate, making your body consume more calories overall. Your body surely consumes a few calories processing suppers. This is named the thermal impact of nourishment. By and large, TEF utilizes around 10% of your complete calorie consumption. Nonetheless, what is important is the absolute number of calories you expend, not what number of suppers you eat. Eating six 500-calorie dinners has a similar impact as eating three 1,000-calorie suppers. Given a normal TEF of 10%, you'll consume 300 calories in the two cases.

Various investigations exhibit that expanding or diminishing dinner recurrence doesn't influence complete calories consumed.

Eating Often Diminishes Hunger

A few people accept that occasional eating forestalls yearnings and exorbitant appetite. However, the proof is blended. Albeit a few investigations propose that eating increasingly visit dinners prompts decreased yearning, different examinations have discovered no impact or even expanded appetite levels.

One investigation that thought about eating three or six high-protein meals every day found that eating three dinners decreased yearning all the more successfully. All things considered; reactions may rely upon the person. In the event that regular eating lessens your yearnings, it's most likely a smart thought. All things considered, there's no proof that eating or eating more often reduces hunger for everybody.

Visit Dinners Can Assist You with Shedding Pounds

Since eating all the more as often as possible doesn't support your digestion, it moreover doesn't have any impact on weight reduction. In reality, an examination in 16 grown-ups with stoutness thought about the impacts of eating 3 to 6 meals per day and found no distinction in weight, fat misfortune, or craving.

A few people guarantee that eating frequently makes it harder for them to hold fast to a healthy diet. Nevertheless, on the off chance that you find that eating all the more frequently makes it simpler for you to eat less calories and less lousy nourishment, don't hesitate to stay with it.

Irregular Fasting Causes You to Lose Muscle

A few people accept that when you fast, your body begins consuming muscle for fuel. In spite of the fact that this occurs with eating less junk food when all is said and done, no proof shows that it happens more with irregular fasting than with different strategies. Then again, consider demonstrating that irregular fasting is better for keeping up bulk. Strikingly, irregular fasting is well known among many bodybuilders, who find that it keeps up muscle close by a low muscle to fat ratio.

Irregular Fasting is Awful for Your Wellbeing

While you may have heard bits of gossip that irregular fasting hurts your wellbeing, exams have uncovered that it instead has several impressive medical advantages. For instance, it changes your quality of articulation identified with life span and resistance and has been appeared to draw out life expectancy in creatures.

It additionally has significant advantages for metabolic wellbeing, for example, it improves insulin sensitivity along with diminishing oxidative pressure, irritation, and coronary illness chance. It might likewise support cerebrum wellbeing by raising degrees of mind inferred neurotrophic factor (BDNF). This is a hormone that may secure against melancholy and different other states of mind.

Various fantasies get propagated about intermittent fasting and feast recurrence. Be that as it may, a large number of these bits of gossip are not valid. For instance, eating smaller, increasingly visit dinners doesn't support your digestion or assist you with shedding pounds. In addition, discontinuous fasting is a long way from undesirable and may offer various advantages. It's essential to counsel sources or do a little research before forming a hasty opinion about your metabolism and general wellbeing.

Myths about intermittent fasting

Issues that are not popular can be misunderstood with a lot of misconceptions and myths surrounding them. Intermittent fasting is one such issue. Many people with half-baked information suddenly become experts on the topic and are always willing to give advice to anyone willing to listen. This chapter debunks some of these myths. It doesn't matter how long a false premise is considered correct, once the evidence is present, the error is exposed and wise people will know to stick with the facts.

Intermittent Fasting Is Unsafe for Older Adults

Anyone can engage in intermittent fasting as long as they do not have any medical conditions and are not pregnant or lactating. Of course, our bodies do not all have the same tolerance levels even in people that look exactly alike. If one or more people respond negatively to intermittent fasting because they are advanced in age and are women, it does not mean that another women in her 50s will react the same way.

There is no doubt that intermittent fasting is not meant for everyone. Fasting is not safe for children because they need all the food they can get for continual development. Fasting in itself is not an issue for older people – any adult can fast.

You Gain Weight as You Age

A myth is a combination of facts and falsehood. This is a typical example of that. It is saying that growing older means your metabolism will slow down and your body will not burn or use up calories as fast as when you were younger. However, weight gain in older adults is not a given. The key to keeping your body performing optimally is to develop and maintain healthy habits such as fasting intermittently, drinking enough water, reducing stress levels, and getting adequate exercise.

Your Metabolism Slows Down During Fasting

This myth represents one of those big misunderstandings I mentioned earlier. The difference between calorie restriction and deliberately choosing when to take in calories is huge. Intermittent fasting does not necessarily limit calorie intake neither does it make you starve. It is when a person starves or under-eats that changes occur in their metabolic rate. But there is no change whatsoever in your metabolism when you delay eating for a few hours by fasting intermittently.

You Will Get Fat If You Skip Breakfast

"Breakfast is the most important meal of the day!" This is one of the more popular urban myths about intermittent fasting. It is in the same category with the myths, *"Santa doesn't give you presents if you're naughty!"* and *"carrots give you night vision."* Some people will readily point to a relative or friend who is fat because they don't eat breakfast. But the question is: are they fat because they don't eat breakfast? Or do they skip breakfast because they are fat and want to reduce their calorie intake?

The best way to collect unbiased data when conducting scientific studies is through randomized controlled trials (RTC). After a careful study of 13 different RTCs on the relationship between weight gain and eating or skipping breakfast, researchers from Melbourne, Australia found that both overweight and normal-weight participants who ate breakfast gained more weight than participants who skipped breakfast. The researchers also found that there's a higher rate of calorie consumption later in the day in participants who ate breakfast. This puts a hole in the popular notion that skipping breakfast will make people overeat later in the day (Harvard Medical School, 2019).

The truth is, there is nothing spectacular about eating breakfast, as far as weight management is concerned. There is limited scientific evidence disproving or supporting the idea that breakfast influences weight. Instead, studies only show that there is no difference in weight loss or gain when one eats or skips breakfast.

Exercise is Harmful to Older Adults Especially While Fasting

No, it is not harmful to exercise while fasting. And no, exercise is not harmful to older adults, whether they are fasting or not. On the contrary, exercising during your fasting window helps to burn stored fats in the body. When you perform physical activities after eating, your body tries to burn off new calories that are ingested from your meal. But when you exercise on an empty, or nearly empty stomach, your body burns fats that are already stored and keeps you fit.

What is harmful to older adults is not engaging in exercises at all. A lack of exercise or adequate physical activity in older adults is linked to diabetes, heart disease, and obesity among other health conditions.

Researchers from Harvard Medical School demonstrated in a landmark study that frail and old women could regain functional loss through resistance exercise (Harvard Medical School, 2007). For ten weeks, participants from a nursing home (100 women aged between 72 and 98) performed resistance exercises three times a week. At the end of 10 weeks, the participants could walk faster and further, climb more stairs, and lift a great deal more weight than their inactive counterparts. Also, a 10-year study of healthy aging by researchers with the MacArthur Study of Aging in America found that older adults (people between 70 and 80 years) can become physically fit whether or not they have been exercising at their younger age. The bottom line is, as long as you can move the muscles in your body, do it because it is safe and will only help you live a better and longer life.

Eating Frequently Reduces Hunger

There is mixed scientific evidence in this regard. Some studies show that eating frequently reduces hunger in some people. On the other hand, other studies show the exact opposite. Interestingly, at least one study shows no difference in the frequency of eating and how it influences hunger (US National Library of Medicine, 2013). Eating can help some people get over cravings and excessive hunger, but there is no evidence to prove that it applies to everyone.

"You Can't Teach an Old Dog New Tricks"

The brain never stops learning. Neither does it stop developing at any age. New neural pathways are created when a person learns something new at any age. With continued repetition, the neural pathways become stronger until the behavior is habitual. Older people are often more persistent and have a higher motivation than younger people when it comes to learning new things. Learning should be a lifelong pursuit and not an activity reserved for young people.

Don't allow anyone to convince you into believing that it is too late to learn new eating habits because you are in your golden years or are approaching it. It doesn't matter if you've never tried fasting, you can still train your brain to make fasting a habit even in old age. Start small, make it a natural occurrence in everyday life, and repeat until you get used to it. Your positive results, such as glowing skin and improved energy, will motivate you to make it into a lifestyle.

You Must Lose Weight during Intermittent Fasting

This myth is rooted in the hype that intermittent fasting has received in recent years. Unless done correctly, intermittent fasting may not yield weight loss benefits. For you to experience any significant loss in weight, you must ensure that you eat healthily during your eating window. Equally, it is important to stick to the fasting schedule. If you keep cheating and adjusting your fasting window to favor more eating time, or you overeat during the eating window to compensate for lost meals, your chances of losing weight will be greatly diminished.

Your Body Will Go Into "Starvation Mode" If You Practice Intermittent Fasting

This myth is based on the misconception of what the starvation mode is and what triggers it. First of all, starvation is when your body senses that there is a significant drop in energy supply and reduces your metabolic rate. In simple terms, it is a reduction in the rate at which your body burns fat as a lack of food. This is an automatic response to conserve energy. It makes sense to reduce energy consumption if there is little to no supply of further energy coming from meals. In other words, if you stay away from food for too long, your body activates the starvation mode and significantly stops any further loss of body fat.

Having said that, intermittent fasting does not trigger the starvation mode. Instead, intermittent fasting helps to increase your metabolic activities. Meaning, your body can burn more fat when you fast for short periods. Starvation mode is only triggered when you engage in prolonged fasting for over 48 hours, a practice I do not recommend for older adults.

An Aging Skin Is Better Taken Care of with Anti-Aging Cream

This is not necessarily true. Brown spots, sagging skin, and wrinkles can indeed be reversed using expensive creams and topical treatments, especially if a dermatologist prescribes them. These topical products exfoliate the top layer of your skin and make them appear smoother. However, the result (clear, smooth skin) is only a temporary effect.

A better way to look younger, without any side effects, is by activating autophagy. Engaging in mild stress-inducing activities, such as intermittent fasting and exercising, are the way. One key element to maintaining healthy skin is quenching your skin's thirst. Not drinking enough water can damage skin causing it to become dry, blemished, and lead to wrinkles. Drinking adequate amounts of water every day is the best approach to successfully "take the years off."

Fasting Deprives Your Brain of Adequate Dietary Glucose

Some people believe that your brain will underperform if you don't eat enough food rich in carbohydrates. This myth is rooted in the notion that your brain uses only glucose as its fuel. Your brain doesn't use only dietary glucose for fuel. Some very low-carb diets can cause your body to produce ketone bodies from high-fat foods. Your brain can function well on ketone bodies. Continuous, intermittent fasting coupled with exercise can trigger the production of ketone bodies. Additionally, your body can also use a process known as gluconeogenesis to produce the sugar needed by your brain. This means that your body can effectively produce it on its own without you feeding it only carbs.

Intermittent fasting does not interfere with brain function or its fuel and energy needs. However, because intermittent fasting is not suitable for everyone, if you feel shaky, dizzy, or extremely fatigued during fasting, consider talking with your doctor or reducing your fasting window.

Intermittent Fasting Will Make Older Adults Lose Their Muscle

First of all, it is stereotypical and largely incorrect to think of older people as frail. Frailty is not limited to older adults and is a generalization of old age. For example, younger people can become frail if they suffer from a disabling chronic disease or have a poor diet. Scientists studied data from almost half a million people and found that middle-aged adults as young as 37 show signs of frailty (Mail Online, 2018).

Secondly, intermittent fasting does not lead to muscle loss in young or older people. On the contrary, fasting intermittently can help you maintain better muscle mass. It is, therefore, not surprising that intermittent fasting is a common practice among bodybuilders to help them maintain muscle mass.

All Fasting Outcomes Are the Same

This myth is rooted in the assumption that everyone has exactly the same physical and chemical makeup. No two individuals are the same regardless of how identical they appear to be. Age, existing medical conditions, body types and size, and level of commitment to the practice are among the many factors that can significantly influence your results.

A woman who fasts for twelve hours twice a week is likely to have a different result from another woman who fasts for 16 hours four times a week. Even when people follow the same fasting regimen, their results will still vary and that is to be expected. Fasting results are not typical in any way. Thinking fasting results should all be the same can lead to a weird frame of mind full of unnecessary comparison, pushing yourself too hard, or giving up too soon because your results don't look anything like that of other women you've seen.

Frequently Asked Questions About Intermittent Fasting

Can I have coffee?

Yes, you can have black coffee, water, and plain steeped tea.

Can I add cream/sugar/milk in my coffee?

The goal of fasting is not to add calories, so the answer is no; you should not add anything to your coffee. However, I have heard of cases in which intermittent fasters add less than 50 calories to their coffee. They have claimed to still be successful with intermittent fasting. I have heard this does not affect their fasted state, but keep in mind all individuals are not created equal. I would not recommend adding anything to your coffee. However, if adding something to your coffee still makes this a good change for the goal you have for yourself, then give it a try.

Does intermittent fasting work well with veganism, paleo, keto, vegetarianism, or any other styles of eating?

Yes, the beauty of intermittent fasting is that it can be combined with any style of eating unless otherwise directed by a medical professional. You can turn your style of eating into the 16:8 method with ease, as this change does not restrict or state the style/types of food you eat; it is specifically based on the timing of your eating.

Is there an alternative to the 16:8 method if I cannot initially fast 16 hours and want to work my way up to 16?

Yes, especially for women, it is recommended that if women cannot or are not willing to do a 16 hour fast, they can start with a 14-hour fasting window and 10-hour feeding window. This is recommended for women, but men can start here if needed as well. Once the 14 hours are mastered, you can then work your way up to the 16:8 method.

Can I have a cheat meal?

You can technically eat what you want when intermittent fasting; there are no food group restrictions. Therefore, there is no cheat meal to have unless you have decided that you have put yourself on some restrictive meals/foods to not indulge in. If this is the case, then yes, but I recommend to always eat in moderation.

What are some healthy snack foods to eat on the go during my feeding window?

Pepperoni slices, fruit, veggie tray, Skinny Pop popcorn individual bags (unless you will always measure the servings before consuming), turkey/beef jerky, individual peanut butter cups, whole-grain cereal, almond milk, eggs, rice cakes, nuts (individual bags), hummus, and more.

I am too hungry during my fasting window; what should I do?

Be patient, and wait for your body to adapt to this change. This may take some time. For some, this change occurs fast; for others, it may take a week or so, but this depends on how you were eating before starting this new lifestyle. According to Collier in 2013, your body is still adjusting to how it was functioning before and is fighting you to get back to that way, as most people were eating more frequently and maybe even more meals or snacks during the day. Eventually, you will not feel this way. You will adapt to your feeding and fasting windows, and the urge to eat or the thought of starving will become milder and milder until it goes away.

Why am I not losing fat faster, like other people are?

It is more than likely a combination of not eating the appropriate portions when you are eating and/or not preparing to eat the right food choices. Although fat and weight loss can still happen, it's more frequent and visible when the appropriate food choices and portions are selected and prepared.

How can I stay full longer?

Eat more fiber and drink more water.

Do I have to eat low carb?

No, you can eat whatever you want during your feeding window. However, I recommend eating proportionately and choosing healthier food options. Instead of white bread, choose whole-grain bread. Instead of white rice, choose brown rice. Instead of anything with high fructose corn syrup, scratch it off. Instead of canned fruit, eat fresh fruit.

Should I exercise in the fasted state?

You can, but it is not required. It is also not recommended on heavy lifting days.

What if I am on medications and must eat with my morning medications?

In this case, you would need to make your feeding window begin at whatever time you take your meds. I would recommend taking your meds as late as you can in the mornings but get authorization of your plan from a medical professional.

Should I discuss this with my medical professional before beginning the change?

Yes, you should always discuss diet changes with a medical professional before you begin.

Why should one start intermittent fasting?

The number-one reason for starting this diet plan is to lose weight without changing one's diet to an extreme level. With this diet plan, you are free to retain your body's muscle mass and stay lean. This is possible because IF reduces belly fat as the diet progresses. As this diet plan requires little change and no complicated routines, it is an effective and simple way to lose weight.

Is skipping breakfast considered unhealthy for the body?

This is a myth that most people think of as being true. This stereotype must be avoided. Some say that getting up and having breakfast helps the body get the energy it needs for the whole day. That might be true, but if you are following a healthy diet for the rest of your meals, skipping breakfast should not affect your lifestyle. It may take some time to get used to skipping a meal after you wake up with an empty stomach, but that will help the absorptive state take place to detoxify the body and clean your insides.

Is it okay to take supplements with an intermittent fasting regimen?

Yes, you can consume those as well. However, you may need to check on certain supplements. Some of them may work better than others. For instance, fat-soluble vitamins will be more effective with your meals during eating hours. Choose them over other types of supplements.

Some experts recommend consuming BCAAs (branched-chain amino acids) before working out while fasting. This way, the body stays in a fasting state but gets the protein to have a vigorous workout routine. It ensures that you have high stamina and energy to work out for a longer duration without tiring out.

Will intermittent fasting affect one's metabolism?

No, it will not affect the metabolism if the fasting period is short-term. However, studies have shown that fasting for longer periods of time (like two or three days) can reduce metabolism.

Intermittent fasting focuses on short-term fasting goals, so it should not affect your metabolism. Instead, it will boost it for more effective processing.

Can a child fast?

No, it would be a bad idea for a child to fast. In a child's case, skipping breakfast can cause a lack of growth hormones in their body, and he or she might not develop normally. The child may also lack proper brain function if he or she follows intermittent fasting for a prolonged period.

How to Deal with the Side Effects of Intermittent Fasting

This chapter will delve into the possible negative side effects of fasting intermittently. Some people who swear by this practice may not be willing to admit that there are unpleasant side effects of fasting intermittently. However, that would be myopic and withholding vital information.

Having said that, it is important to point out that the general downsides of intermittent fasting are common to all women regardless of age. While women of child-bearing age might have effects on their reproductive hormones, post-menopausal women or older women may not need to worry about reproduction. Although, they may experience frequent changes in their moods, difficulty in sleeping, and occasional headaches.

After a comprehensive review of several scientific studies on women's health, fasting, and aging, researchers weren't able to find any significant negative effect of intermittent fasting and point to a lack of research on the topic (Journal of Mid-Life Health, 2016). These types of scientific reviews are very useful for getting unbiased information that gives you a broader picture of several results from different related studies performed over many years. Comprehensive reviews cut down prejudices often associated with smaller studies that may have been sponsored by special interest groups. Overall, scientific studies show encouraging results in different aspects of women's health including mental health, physical health, and weight loss. That is not to say, there are no negative side effects of intermittent fasting. It only means that the negative side effects of intermittent fasting are common to women of all ages, both pre and post-menopausal women, and depend largely on the individual woman.

With that being said, not everyone who practices intermittent fasting will have a negative side effect. These differ from person to person. The important thing is being aware of these negative side effects and learning how to handle them if they occur. Also, remember that most of the off-putting effects of intermittent fasting don't last beyond the first few days. Within a week or two, your body would have adjusted to your new eating schedule and any negative effects will gradually subside until things feel back to normal. So it is important to allow your body some time to adjust instead of trying intermittent fasting for one or two days and throwing in the towel.

Here is how to deal with some of the common negative side effects you are likely to encounter as you start your new eating habits.

Hunger

One of the first and most obvious results of fasting is hunger. This side effect is difficult because going without food longer than your body is conditioned to will result in an uncomfortable desire to eat anything. All your life, you have programmed your body to expect food at certain times throughout the day. It would be weird if you suddenly change your eating pattern, and your body accepts the change without putting up a little resistance. If your body doesn't get food at the time it normally does, a hormone called ghrelin – the hunger hormone – will start acting up to remind you that you should supply your body with food. This "acting up", or reminder to eat at your usual time, will continue until your brain convinces ghrelin to accept your new eating schedule. But until then, you will likely feel intense hunger but don't worry, it will pass. You will need to tap into your reserve of mental strength to stay committed to your course.

To effectively handle hunger pangs you should drink more water, or any qualifying beverage on intermittent fasting. Doing so will help to suppress hunger pangs. Quite often, the feeling of hunger is not necessarily an indication that you are hungry. Instead, it might be a slight dip in your blood sugar level – something that water or other non-calorie liquids can take care of.

To help delay hunger on your fasting days or during the fasting window (depending on the type of fasting regimen you choose to follow), ensure that you include adequate amounts of healthy fats, carbs, and proteins in your meals before commencing your fast. Also, during your fast, try to keep your mind off food. Combining low-impact exercises with fasting can help give you the boost you need to go through your day without feeling too uncomfortable. Getting enough sleep will also help you throughout the day. There is nothing that will upset your day more than lack of sleep at night and then having to fast. That is an open invitation for fatigue and hunger!

Frequent Urination

As with hunger, it is also expected to experience an increase in the number of times you urinate. There is no mystery here as to why this is due to intermittent fasting requiring that you increase your intake of water and other liquids to stay hydrated. This will in turn increase the frequency of urination. Keep drinking your water and don't avoid bathroom visits. Holding itfor too long can weaken your bladder muscles and trying not to drink water will soon make you dehydrated and provide the next side effect – both bad!

Headaches

Intermittent fasting can make your blood sugar take a nosedive. This introduces stress on your body, your brain will release stress hormones, and you will likely experience some degree of headache. Dehydration can lead to headaches during intermittent fasting as your body is telling you it lacks adequate water.

To reduce the occurrence of headaches, try to minimize stress on your body. It is okay to exercise during fasting, but excessive exercise can trigger a large amount of stress. Also, try to keep your body hydrated at all times by drinking enough water. However, don't chug water in a rush and don't drink water excessively. Too much water can result in an imbalance in your mineral and body water ratio.

Cravings

It is normal to experience more cravings for food during your fasting window. This is a biological and psychological response to the feeling of deprivation that is often associated with going without food. Because your body is trying to get glucose, you might notice that you crave more sugar or carbohydrates. These cravings don't mean that you are less committed to your goals. Rather, cravings happen to remind you that you are human. Even ardent practitioners of intermittent fasting experience cravings from time to time.

When food cravings start, remind yourself of your goal and distract yourself from food-related topics. Keep your mind engrossed with other non-food-related activities such as hobbies, talking a walk in nature, or taking a nap. During your eating window, you can treat yourself to a healthy bite of what you crave to minimize the intensity of the craving or longing. Remind yourself during your fasting window that you will soon eat what you long for, so there's no need to dwell on it or give it too much thought when it is not yet time to eat. Remind your body that you are no longer a teenager or a young adult. You have had lots of experience in curbing your cravings, and this case is not an exception.

Heartburn, Bloating, and Constipation

Occasionally, heartburn can occur when your stomach produces acids for digestion of your food, but there is no food present in the stomach to be digested. Bloating and constipation usually go hand in hand and can also occur in some cases. Together, these two can make you feel very uncomfortable.

Drinking adequate amounts of water can reduce the risk of heartburn, bloating, and constipation. Heartburns can also be minimized by cutting down on spicy foods during your eating window. If you experience heartburn during intermittent fasting, here's something you can try before going to sleep. Prop yourself up when you lie down to sleep. However, don't use pillows to prop yourself as that will put more pressure on your stomach and increase the discomfort. Use a specially designed wedge or use a 6-inch block, or something similar, to elevate your head as you lie down. Doing this will make gravity minimize the backward flow of your stomach contents into your gullet. Propping yourself this way should bring you relief from heartburn. However, if heartburn, bloating, and constipation persist, consult your doctor immediately.

Binging

Eating a large amount as soon as the fasting window is over is usually associated with first-timers to intermittent fasting. The intense hunger of fasting can drive you to eat in a hurry when breaking your fast, and you can end up overeating. In some cases, binging can be a result of a simple misunderstanding of the basics of intermittent fasting. A person may assume that they can eat as much as they want in the eating window since the no-eating window will take care of the calories. This misunderstanding can deprive you of gaining any significant benefits that come with fasting intermittently, especially if you are looking to shed some weight. Binging or overeating in your eating window will reverse all the hard work you put in during the fast.

To avoid binging, ensure that the sizes and type of meals are planned well ahead of the eating window. Don't start fasting without knowing what portion you are going to consume at the end of the fasting window. Waiting until your eating window to decide what to eat and how much to eat can lead to overeating because your food choices will become largely influenced by how hungry you feel.

Low Energy

Feeling exhausted is a normal part of fasting. Until your body gets used to sourcing its fuel from fat storage, you are likely to experience some decline in your energy levels. Usually, they go back to normal within a couple of days.

To help stay energized, tailor your activities to remain low-key when you first start intermittent fasting. There is no need to push yourself to prove that you are a strong woman. Deciding to practice intermittent fasting is enough proof that you are mentally, emotionally, and physically strong. Since you are not in competition with anyone, it is in your best interest to conserve energy as much as possible. Get a massage, spend time relaxing in bed, or sleeping in if you can. These little activities can go a long way in keeping you energized.

Feeling Cold

Some people experience feeling cold more often during fasting. If you experience this, there is no cause for alarm. It might be a result of the drop in your blood sugar level. Usually, blood flow to your internal fat storage is increased during fasting. As a result of this increase, your fat is moved to parts of your body where it needs to be used as energy. This can make other parts of your body that have less fat storage experience cold. If you feel cold in your fingers or toes, it is your body doing its fat burning process for your own good.

To help reduce the cold, put on layers of clothes, stay in warm places, drink hot coffee or tea (with no calories), or take a hot shower. It is important to keep in mind that feeling cold is just a result of intermittent fasting and does not mean you are ill.

So avoid the urge to self-medicate. If the cold feeling persists even in your non-fasting days or in your eating window, consult your doctor.

Mood Swing

Imagine the following combinations. Stress on your body caused by the dip in your blood sugar. Your hormones are going berserk from the various reactions going on in your body as a result of not eating normally, or on schedule. The lethargic feeling from lack of food, hunger, and cravings constantly telling you to eat. Not being able to socialize with others freely because of your new eating pattern meaning you can't wine and dine at social events if it is outside your eating window! All of these can lead to a psychological state of feeling annoyed or irritated.

The surest way to minimize mood swings resulting from intermittent fasting is to deliberately keep your attention off issues that set you on edge and focus on what you are doing and what makes you happy. The more you keep your mind wrapped up in gratitude and appreciation, the better you will feel. So, during your fasting window, be deliberate about engaging in things that lift your spirits and keep your mind on happy and productive thoughts.

Bottom Line

Intermittent fasting is a lifestyle regimen that is safe for older practitioners. It is a medical intervention that can bring about improvements in many aspects of a woman's health. However, it is not suitable for every person. If you notice that you have any severe negative reactions to intermittent fasting, it is in your best interest to desist at once and consult your doctor. No rule makes it compulsory to complete a fast once you begin. You can absolutely break in the middle of your fasting window (even if it is just for that day) if you can no longer endure unpleasant side effects and try again at a later time.

While it is okay to give your body a few weeks to get used to your new eating pattern, it is also crucial to pay close attention to what your body is telling you. Thankfully, as an older woman with experience, you can tell when something works for you or not. You know when you can commit to something and when you can't find the motivation to follow through. I believe that, as a woman with a tremendous wealth of experience, you will find the strength to stick to your resolve within reason.

Foods to Eat

Every diet comes with a limited list of ingredients or a limited calorie scale to remain in. However, intermittent fasting neither has a calorie limit, unless you pick the 5:2 method of fasting, nor does it contain any list of ingredients that are allowed or forbidden. Only the 5:2 method of intermittent fasting is limited to 500-600 calories per day for 2 days.

Intermittent fasting allows you to eat anything you like in your eating windows. There are no guidelines, restrictions, or lists!

However, since this is a diet and you have started intermittent fasting for a reason, be it to lose weight, gain better lifespan, getting hold of your eating habit, combating diseases like cancer, type-2 diabetes, or any other chronic diseases; eating in a healthy manner is always advised.

The fitness experts and other researchers would suggest sticking to whole foods. This does not mean processed food is forbidden in intermittent fasting, but you need to know what foods are good for your body and which are doing damage to your body and then decide whether or not you would want processed food in your menu!

Processed food is usually packed with added flavors, sugar, and chemicals to keep it preserved for months. These added flavors, sugar, and chemicals do harm to our body. They may taste good, but we need to weigh the taste with the damage it is indulging upon us. Once you have made the call of cutting down processed food altogether from your menu, you will find many substitutes that are organic and have no added flavors or hidden chemicals in them. The worst thing these hidden chemicals can do to our body is make us lethargic and fatty.

Switching to non-processed foods may take a while, but once you get used to it, you will find it much easier to continue intermittent fasting.

For example, a peanut butter sandwich is something we all love for breakfast, but store-bought peanut butter has many preservatives in them. You can, instead, simply make it at home with 3 ingredients. If you have a good food processor, it will take less than a minute to make peanut butter at home. The store-bought peanut butter also costs you more. Store-bought ketchup is another example; this too can be made at home with very few ingredients and without harmful chemicals. Whatever food you are using every day for your menu, try to make it at home without any chemicals. This way you do not have to compromise on the taste and you will not damage your body either.

Processed food also contributes to gaining weight. If you are wanting to lose weight, this is another good reason to avoid processed food altogether. Sometimes the ingredients listed on the processed food's label is in their code names and people may not always know what code stands for what ingredient! This can be very tricky when you are a vegetarian or trying to avoid certain foods. For instance, Muslims do not eat pork and many foods contain pig fat in them. The ingredient list does not always say "pig fat" in it, rather it gives away a code specified for "pig fat". If you leave out processed food altogether, you will not have to worry about what code stands for what which can lead to accidentally eat something that you didn't want to swallow.

If losing weight is your main target when you start intermittent fasting, then of course you should only stick to a well-balanced diet. A diet where every nutritious fruit and vegetable, meat, seafood, and carbohydrate is present! You need to design your meal plan accordingly. Choose food that is good to increase energy level, lowers lethargy, and does not leave you feeling full. Intermittent fasting should leave you feeling light and good about yourself. If you feel full and blotted, then you are doing something wrong and you need to change your menu.

It is essential to combine your proteins with high fiber food to make your digestion process easier. As you are fasting, you may notice some changes in your digestion system and your bowel movement. This is natural as your eating pattern has changed. Do not be alarmed but be aware if some food is not working for you during intermittent fasting, you may need to change it and adopt some new recipes with new ingredients. High fiber food is easy to digest but do not consume too much of it as it may cause diarrhea. The eating pattern should be balanced.

Below is a list of a few ingredients that should be on the menu.

Water

As mentioned earlier, being hydrated is essential during any diet and particularly during intermittent fasting when you are refraining from food, it is crucial not to become dehydrated. You will need to drink at least 8 glasses of water every day. Make a routine of drinking water every hour. You can also fill up a 2-liter water bottle with water and keep it somewhere you can see so you get a reminder of drinking water every time you look at it. Many people get gestational problems when they drink too much water. But the truth is if you do not drink enough water, your health would decay and your gestational problems would only increase. Dehydration also triggers many other problems in the human body like jaundice, fatigue, headache, and lightheadedness. The last thing you would want in an intermittent fasting period is these health issues.

If you cannot drink water, try drinking fruit juices, vegetable juice, coconut water, etc. Smoothies are another option but they may have so many sweetening agents that only one glass of it should be enough for a day. If you are doing the 5:2 method of intermittent fasting, then leaving out the smoothie is recommended as it probably contains lots of calories.

Fish

Fish is a super-brain food. It improves your cognition power. Intermittent fasting may cause dizziness and sometimes messes with the power of your cognition. Therefore, eating a lot of fish during intermittent fasting is a good idea. Fish is filled with Vitamin D and Omega 3 amino acids. There are not many foods where you can find Vitamin D. Vitamin D is very good for the heart, our skin, and our growth. Fish has other healthy fats too. So to fill you up with lots of nutrition, fish is a great choice.

You can eat any fish; there is no particular suggestion here. However, researches have shown fishes like salmon and tuna have many benefits and are eaten throughout the world widely. Salmon and tuna can be found in cans too. If you live in a place where fresh salmon and tuna are not available, you can go for the canned ones. However, read the labels and see if any preservatives used in the can are particularly harmful to you or not.

Some people cannot eat fish, no matter if you make a fish curry, fish fry, fish soup, or fish chowder, they simply cannot handle the smell. In that case, try making fish kebabs. They taste excellent and they do not have any smell of fish. If you do not tell someone the kebabs are made out of fish, they probably would not even guess it is because of their delicious taste.

Apple

We know the saying, "An apple a day keeps the doctor away".

This was said for a good reason. Apples contain many healthy nutrients like anti-oxidant, mineral, magnesium, fiber, etc. It also gives you good digestion and provides you with healthy-looking skin. You can eat an apple fresh or make a jam out of it and use it to make sandwiches. You can also make pancakes and other desserts using apples. An apple smoothie or juice is also quite delicious.

Banana

Bananas are very high in calories and some people rule out bananas during a weight loss diet. But a banana is very good for the health too. It keeps you energized and fills your tummy for a long time.

Adding banana into your breakfast and smoothies is another good option. Banana bread and banana cake is also a very tasty and healthier option for baking. Whenever you have very ripe bananas or leftover bananas, make banana bread or banana cake, it will serve you well.

Seafood

Seafood like clam, squid, calamari, and snail are very good for your health. Like fish, they are high in omega 3 and vitamin D. They are light in texture and require very little cooking and prepping time in the kitchen. Seafood gives you instant energy and keeps you feeling active for about six hours. Try adding seafood to your menu every other day.

Fiber rich vegetables

Fiber is essential for our body and when you are doing intermittent fasting, it may mess with your digestive system. Most people get constipation due to not getting enough liquid or fiber. The last thing you would want during intermittent fasting is getting constipated. To prevent constipation, relying on supplements, syrups or other herbal medicines is not always wise as most of these products have their own side effects. If you use them for a long period of time, your body will reject them and it may cause your constipation problem to get worse.

A good solution for constipation is consuming a good amount of high-fiber foods. Vegetables are a great source of high-fiber.

Vegetables like broccoli, cabbage, green beans, Brussels sprout, spinach, basil leaves, cauliflower, carrots, etc. are very fiber enriching. They can be cooked in a variety of ways and to add diversity to your menu, try out new recipes every now and then. The key to eating healthy is to keep trying new things in the kitchen. One cauliflower can be used in a variety of creative and tasty ways. It can be stir-fried, made into curry, incorporated in an omelet, make a pizza crust, substituted for rice if you ground it, baked as a whole, etc. If you try new recipes, the vegetable of your choosing will taste differently and you will not feel bored of eating healthy food either.

Vegetables like broccoli are a super food. It has so many health benefits. Many people do not like the taste or the smell of broccoli. In that case, be creative in the kitchen and try making broccoli soup with mushroom, or make a stir-fry of broccoli and beef, baked broccoli with cheese on top tastes great as well.

Avocado

Avocado is one such fruit that needs to be mentioned separately to emphasize its value. One avocado is enough to keep you going for 6 hours straight. You will not feel any hunger pangs or feel lightheaded afterwards. It is, of course, one of the highest calorie foods, so you may wonder if you can eat it during a weight loss project, but research has shown it contains good protein, which is essential to burn body fat. It keeps you feeling full for a long time; therefore, you do not eat other junk food or snack for a while. This way, you are refraining from eating and it contributes to losing weight.

Avocado is considered to be a green gem; it can be eaten by itself when it is perfectly ripe. You can make it as a salad with goat cheese, mashed or in a smoothie, and you can also make delicious dips with it. Adding avocado slices to your sandwiches also uplifts their nutrition value.

Potatoes

Unlike other diets, intermittent fasting has no restrictions or limitations on carbohydrates. So if you are a fan of potatoes, you are in luck. Fitness experts suggest that eating potatoes during intermittent fasting is good for you. They are the ultimate comfort food in any region and with a large productivity value, potatoes can be found anywhere in the world at any time of the year. They are rather cheap and are considered among the most satiating foods.

Many countries eat potatoes as their staple food. Countries that eat rice occasionally, make mashed potato every day. So this shows how fulfilling the food is. Of course, you cannot eat French fries, potato croutons, potato falafel, potato noodles, or potato chips and think that you are eating healthy food. You need to make proper dishes like mashed potatoes, potato soup, potato curry, or baked potatoes etc. Store bought packed potato chips are one of the worse junk foods you can eat, especially during a diet. They make your belly bloated, give you bad gas problems, and make you feel lethargic etc.

Legumes and Beans

While many diets avoid legumes and beans altogether due to their carbohydrate level, intermittent fasting encourages enjoying a bowl of legumes and beans in chili every now and then. They are very good for your health and contain few calorie, keeping you feeling full for a long time. A healthy diet should have a balance of every type of food and legumes are one of them. Try to consume legumes and beans at least 3 times a week or more; doing so will help you reduce body fat and give you a good eating pattern. Eating junk is always worse than eating calorie-packed foods that are natural.

Legumes and beans can be added to so many recipes. Mexican chili is the first thing that may pop into all of our heads, but they can be used for many other recipes like soups, stews, curries, or even roasted by themselves. If you are craving snacks, try roasting lentils, chickpeas, or beans with some salt and pepper. You have a good homemade snack ready within 10 minutes which has no artificial flavorings.

You can make amazing dips and guacamole using chickpeas. They can be boiled and eaten with a pinch of salt and pepper and a drizzle of lemon juice. Lentil soup is one of the most comforting foods ever during a winter. So there are many good healthy options out there.

Oats

Oats are another super food and among the highest consumed breakfast items around the world. Filled with all the good nutrients, oats are high-fiber and help with digestion. They are a natural remedy for constipation and help combat many diseases as well.

Oats have a fallacy that they are a boring food with no taste. This is wrong and you would be surprised how many variations you can create with oats in the kitchen. To name a few, you can make porridge, pancakes, pudding, burgers, stew, paella, tortillas etc. Oats are usually consumed with sweeteners but taste good when you make them savory.

Nuts and Seeds

Nuts are a good choice to munch on during any diet and uphold numerous nutrition values. Nuts like cashews, almonds, Brazil nuts, peanuts, pistachios, and walnuts etc. are considered very good for the health as they contain non-saturated fat. Many think since nuts are high in fat that they may contribute in gaining weight. But non-saturated fat actually helps reduce body fat and supplies you energy and keeps you active for a long time. The benefit of almonds is very high. Soak them for 30 minutes, peel the skin off and munch away. They will give you instant energy. Making a homemade nutty bar using these nuts is a good option for snacking. The store-bought ones come with many added flavorings and sweetening agents that may trigger weight gain.

Pumpkin and sunflower seeds are very good for the health. Black cumin seeds are another super food you must incorporate into your everyday life; they combat diabetes, cancer, gestational problems, and inflammation. Many people roast the seeds lightly and munch on them anytime they can. The smell and the flavor are rather strong, so if you think you cannot eat them by themselves because of the bitterness, you can add a spoon of honey or a date. Adding natural sweetening agents will remove the bitter taste. You can also add black cumin seeds to stir-fries and curries. People living in Asia, particularly in India, Bangladesh, Pakistan, and Sri Lanka use black cumin seeds in their curries and stir-fries. Some even add them to croutons and tortillas.

Dried Fruits

Dried fruits serve miraculously for providing instant energy and are filled with good nutrients. Dried fruits like dates, figs, plums, cherries, and apricots etc. are not harvested everywhere in the world, therefore, the need to make them dry came forth. They are pretty close to the fresh thing itself. If you soak the dried fruit for 1 hour or so in water or milk, it becomes softer and much tastier.

Dates and figs are filled with magnesium, potassium, calcium, folic acid, antioxidants, fat, and fiber. Can you think of many fruits that have all those macro-nutritional values together? There are not many! So try to add dates and figs into your daily routine. Whenever you are craving something sweet, bite into a date or a fig. They are high-calorie, so 2 to 4 per day are enough if you want to lose weight. When you are making a smoothie, instead of adding sugar, add 2 dates or 2 figs. It will make your smoothie thicker in texture and the taste would be mind-blowing too.

The good thing about dried food is it can be easily stored at room temperature. It does not require keeping in the refrigerator and will remain good for months if you keep it in a clean and dry place. Since they are dried, they can also be easily carried to your work place or wherever you are traveling.

Probiotics

Since this is an intermittent fasting diet, the chances are very high that you will feel hungry at times and before breaking your fast, you may feel the hunger pangs more than ever. This is natural, but you need to feed your body with enough probiotics to survive the diet itself. If you faint or remain dizzy for the entire period, it will not do you any favors. It will in fact do damage to your body rather than doing it good. So adding probiotic-filled food in your menu is essential. Foods like kraut and kefir are good for the health anyway and during intermittent fasting, they should be regularly consumed. Yogurt is good for digestion and the skin too.

Berries

Berries are high in flavonoid. They work magic for your body and skin. You see how skin products and their commercials always use berries in them. It is done for a reason because berries contribute miraculously to keeping the skin flawless and young.

Berries like blueberries, strawberries, mulberries, and raspberries etc. all are very good for the health and taste good too. You can eat 1 cup of any berry per day without worrying about the calories. Berries taste good anyway, so they can easily be eaten by themselves, but you can incorporate them into pancakes, cakes, smoothies, juices, and some savory items too. Dried berries are also good.

Egg

Egg is a super food, it contains a good amount of fat that is essential for our brain cells. Egg can be incorporated into any meal of the day and is essential for baking. It will keep you energized for 4 hours straight. Intermittent fasting can take a toll on the brain and your cognitive function, so having brain food like egg is always good during when fasting.

Dairy

Dairy items are good for our bone health and mental ability. If you can digest cow or goat milk well, then all is well, but just in case if you cannot, you can try yogurt or milk-produced desserts that are low-calorie. You can also use substitute options like coconut, cashew, almond, and soy milk etc. Oftentimes, people who cannot digest milk in its full form can digest it in milk-based dishes without any hassle. Try making pudding, yogurt, and smoothies with milk and then consume it.

Poultry

As mentioned earlier, intermittent fasting does not restrict the consumption of any food items and meat is something many people love but cannot eat during a diet. With intermittent fasting, you can keep small portions of poultry in your everyday menu. White meat is considered good for health anyway; it does not cause any health related problems like red meat does. Chicken and duck are readily available in any part of the world. For turkey, you may need to search a bit because it is not available everywhere. Different types of birds can also be consumed in limited portions. As your goal is to lose weight or live a healthier life, it is always important to control your portion size.

Whole Grain

Whole grain is ruled out of many diets as they are filled with carbohydrates which trigger obesity, but a little bit of it can actually help you reduce body fat. Whole grain keeps you energized and feeling full for a while, which enables you to avoid eating more often. During fasting, you need food that will allow you to continue working at a good pace. Whole grain contributes to this criterion. Different studies have also shown that it can actually rev up your metabolism system. Rice is one of the most popular grains out there, but there are many other options like farro, kamut, bulgur, millet, spelt, amaranth, and sorghum. It is time to step out of your comfort zone and try out these whole grains to see if they fit into your life well or not.

How to Enjoy a Balanced Diet While on Intermittent Fasting

Eating a balanced diet is much more than simply eating a salad. This is especially true when you are practicing intermittent fasting, as you need to ensure that you are consuming the proper amount of both macronutrients and micronutrients. But what are they? Macronutrients are the fuel your body consumes in a larger number, including protein, fat, and carbohydrates. On the other hand, micronutrients are equally essential but consumed in a smaller quantity, including vitamins, minerals, and phytonutrients found within plants. While a salad may offer you some vegetables, if you don't pair it with plenty of protein and fat, you will be depriving your body of necessary fuel. Not only that, but many people make simple salads with only lettuce, which is low on the nutrition scale. You are much better off consuming a variety of fruits and vegetables to absorb all the micronutrients your body requires. In this chapter, we will examine how you can enjoy a healthy and balanced diet with intermittent fasting.

Salads are a go-to choice for many dieters because they are low in calories and contain vegetables. However, when you are practicing intermittent fasting, you must ensure you consume all the calories and nutrients your body requires during your feeding window, and a simple romaine salad with ranch dressing will not do that. Yet, all salads are not created equal. For instance, you may choose to eat a roasted chicken thigh with a kale salad topped with roasted beets, fresh avocado, toasted almonds, goat cheese, apple, and a rich olive oil vinaigrette. If you make a meal such as this, you will be consuming plenty of protein, healthy fats, and a variety of essential fruits and vegetables. Not only will this meal provide you with the macronutrients and micronutrients your body requires, but it will also leave you full and satisfied for hours to come.

Remember not to focus on low-calorie food, but rather nutrient-dense and satisfying meals. This applies whether you are on a standard healthy diet, or if you are pairing the ketogenic diet with intermittent fasting.

Not only do fruits and vegetables offer you a variety of micronutrients that the body requires, but meat can be quite nutritious, as well. While it is important to enjoy red meat in moderation, it has such a high degree of vitamins and minerals that the occasional serving can be incredibly beneficial. Beef is a prime example of nutritious red meat; 26% of it is protein, which means that for every 100g of meat you eat, you can get 26g of vital protein and amino acids to fuel your body throughout your fast. On average, a serving of beef is considered to be 3oz of meat, which contains 22g of protein in total. While beef may contain saturated fats, which should be consumed in moderation, it also has other important and healthy fats such as oleic acid, which is commonly found in avocados and olives, palmitic acid, and stearic acid.

The micronutrients in beef, meaning vitamins and minerals, are essential for the human body. However, many of these nutrients are not well absorbed from plant-based sources. We may absorb a small number of the vitamins and minerals we eat from a salad or roasted vegetables, but the human body absorbs them much more effectively from meat. Let's have a look at some of the micronutrients found in large number within beef:

- Vitamin B12

- Vitamin B6

- Iron

- Selenium

- Zinc

- Creatine

- Taurine

- Niacin

- Glutathione

As you can see, there are many reasons to consume red meat, as it has many nutrients. Other meats, such as fish, also offer several micronutrients while having less saturated fats that can raise cholesterol. When consuming fish, the best sources are smaller fish that are high in fat. The fat in fish is high in omega-3 fatty acids, which most people in Western countries do not consume enough of. This is detrimental, as when we consume low levels of omega-3 and high levels of omega-6 fats, it causes inflammation and increases the risk of disease. But, by lowering your omega-6 intake and increasing your omega-3 consumption, you can greatly improve your health. Fatty fish such as salmon and sardines are two of your best options.

Try to avoid larger fish options, such as tuna, as the larger the fish, the higher the mercury contamination it contains. This is because larger fish eat smaller fish, thereby increasing their mercury contents, and when you eat these fish, the mercury contamination crosses over to you. Sardines are one of the best options, as they are rich in omega-3 fatty acids and since they are small they contain very little mercury. Sardines are also inexpensive and sold in tin cans, making them stay shelf-stable for long periods. If you purchase bone-in sardines, you can also benefit from an increase in calcium for bone health.

As you can see, both meat and fish have many health benefits. Healthy eating goes beyond eating just fruits and vegetables, but it is about everything you eat. To eat a balanced diet, it is important to choose a balance of healthy proteins, fats, and carbohydrates. Of course, you do not need to consume many carbohydrates, as this is the one fuel source the body does not require through consumption. The ketogenic diet, which is extremely low-carb, can further increase the health benefits you receive through intermittent fasting and boost weight loss. The ketogenic diet can also make intermittent fasting easier, and it prioritizes protein and fat consumption while increasing the production of ketones.

When possible, try to choose grass-fed and organic ingredient options, as these not only don't contain harmful substances, they also provide more nutrition. For instance, studies have found that grass-fed butter contains an average of five times the nutrients of grain-fed butter. This increase of nutrients carries over to everything you eat, whether animal-based or plant-based.

It is okay if you can't afford to buy all your ingredients organic and grass-fed, but when you are able, it is best to budget some of your ingredients to at least be higher quality. The best foods to prioritize as organic and grass-fed include meat, vegetables, and fruits on the dirty dozen list. The dirty dozen list is the foods that contain the highest level of contamination from harmful substances, and therefore are safest to buy organic. This list includes:

- Potatoes

- Spinach

- Tomatoes

- Nectarines

- Grapes

- Pears

- Strawberries

- Cherries

- Peaches

- Celery

- Sweet bell peppers

- Apples

While the ketogenic diet pairs well with intermittent fasting, not everyone chooses to combine the two lifestyles, and that is okay. If you decide to not go on the ketogenic diet, then be sure to prioritize the quality of the carbohydrates you are consuming, as well. You don't want to eat tons of fruit, which is high in glucose and fructose. Fruit is good in moderation, but remember that sugar is sugar, whether it is coming from fruit or cane sugar.

It is best also to choose whole grains rather than processed grains, as the fiber content is higher. This is important, as fiber improves digestive health, allows your body to absorb nutrients better, removes harmful cholesterol from the body, and helps you to remain full and satisfied for longer periods. On the other hand, processed grains that have had most of their fiber removed will spike your blood sugar and in turn, cause a blood sugar crash, making you feel hungry and tired.

When choosing sources of fat, remember that not all fat is created equal. You should prioritize monounsaturated fats such as those in olives, avocados, and nuts. These are the healthiest sources of fats. The second-best source of fat is polyunsaturated fats, which you can find in seeds, walnuts, fish, safflower oil, and soy-based products. The saturated fats found in meats and coconut oil can raise cholesterol and, therefore, should be eaten in moderation. Yes, you can enjoy beef and other meats as they have nutritional benefits, but remember always to prioritize the healthier fats over saturated ones. For instance, instead of eating full-fat meat, you may purchase a lower-fat cut of ground beef and alternatively add fat to your meal with olive oil, avocado oil, or toasted nuts. This will ensure you can both get the nutrients in meat while also prioritizing the best sources of heart-healthy fat.

How Women Over 50 Can Practice Intermittent Fasting Safely

When Not to Fast

There are a few conditions for when intermittent fasting is not advisable.

Pregnant or Breastfeeding

It is highly discouraged to do intermittent fasting when a woman is either pregnant or breastfeeding. Both of these situations require a constant supply of balanced nutrients in the bloodstream and this is impossible to achieve through intermittent fasting. However, balanced diets consumed in your eating periods will still fall short during the fasting window when the only available energy resources are fats. This will not only be harmful to the baby but also to the mother, as all the available resources are put in use for meeting the baby's needs and this deprives the mother of much needed nutrients and energy resources.

Type 1 Diabetics

Type 1 diabetics are another group of people who are widely discouraged from taking part in any form of fasting schedules. This is because in Type 1 diabetes a person is unable to produce any insulin. This makes the blood glucose levels go high because the body needs insulin to process blood glucose. Type 1 diabetics are unequivocally discouraged from intermittent fasting as it is highly risky and dangerous. Since intermittent fasting primarily brings insulin levels down, therefore, we wouldn't want to bring down its levels when they are already low or rather completely absent from the bloodstream. Type 1 diabetics are rightly advised to stay away from intermittent fasting or any fasting schedules for that matter. It is better to be safe than sorry.

Eating Disorders and Underweight

People who have eating disorders of any kind, such as anorexia or bulimia, are discouraged from taking part in intermittent fasting. It is highly inadvisable to put your body through strenuous fasting routines when it is already suffering from the effects of disorderly eating habits. Also, people who are already underweight, which means their body weights fall below the ideal weight for their age and height, are also discouraged from doing intermittent fasting. Not only would it not be ideal, but it would be highly inappropriate and unnecessary to coerce your body into even more restrictive eating habits. If you have a history of eating disorders, fasting of any sort is highly discouraged, as it can be a trigger to prior destructive patterns. There are better suited ways for you to regain and maintain your health, in this case.

Consulting Your Doctor

If you do not fall into any of these categories but are still doubtful of whether you can do intermittent fasting or not, it is always better to consult your doctor before you begin. Tell your doctor your wish to participate in intermittent fasting and place all your health concerns before them. Only when they give you the go ahead, is it proper for you to begin planning your fasts.

Type 2 Diabetes and Intermittent Fasting

Type 2 diabetics are those who are insulin-resistant. Insulin resistance is when your body is producing insulin, but you are unable to make use of it to monitor your blood glucose. To understand it better, there is another way of looking at it.

Imagine if you are used to eating non-stop, round the clock. You are used to munching on snacks or any available food on the go. What this does is keep your insulin levels high all the time. After a certain period of time your body gets used to these elevated levels of insulin. This requires you to produce even more insulin after mealtimes, because your body has in a way, "stopped listening" to the normal levels. This goes on until your body is no longer able to make use of the insulin present in the bloodstream though you are able to produce it.

People with type 2 diabetes have been known to benefit from monitored food intake and regular exercise. This is even truer in cases where intermittent fasting is applied. Type 2 diabetics are able to control their insulin levels and blood glucose levels with the help of intermittent fasting techniques. Obesity and unnatural weight gain are mostly common in people with type 2 diabetes, and this is effectively handled and addressed by participating in intermittent fasting. If you are a type 2 diabetic, talk with your doctor about what type of fasting would suit you. Work with your physician to see what mode of fasting would benefit you most keeping your diabetes and your other health and physical parameters in mind.

Consider Supplementation

Supplementing may be very beneficial and even necessary when fasting to maintain and improve health. This is especially beneficial to women over the age of 50, who may need certain nutrients and minerals even more than others do.

Some essential nutrients and minerals that your body would greatly benefit from like omega-3 or iron may be difficult to get in adequate amounts if you are fasting. For this reason, supplementing them may benefit you in terms of keeping you feeling healthy and energetic, as well as keeping your brain functioning to its full potential. You can take specific nutrients on their own in pill-form, or you can opt for a multivitamin that will include all of the essential vitamins and minerals for overall good health. These vitamins and minerals may differ from those that we looked at in the previous chapter, as those included the vitamins and minerals that are known to induce autophagy. The vitamins included in a multivitamin will be those that are known to promote good overall health and those that are usually obtained through a balanced, whole food diet.

Nutrients You Need and How to Get Them

In this section, we are going to look at the most beneficial nutrients for your body and where/how you can find them when following a specific diet. For women over the age of 50, it is important to ensure that you are getting all of the nutrients that your body needs, especially if you are trying to lose weight or are following a regime that includes fasting. To ensure that your fasting periods are as healthy as possible, supplementation is something that could be considered to ensure that you are feeding your body the nutrients it needs. It is always preferable to get the nutrients you need from whole foods rather than from supplements, but in some cases, when you cannot get everything you need from the foods in your diet alone (especially if you are eating fewer calories), then supplementation is always better than nothing. Below, we will look at some whole food sources as well as some supplements that you may wish to consider.

Omega-3 Fatty Acids

These are essential since they cannot be made in our bodies and must be obtained through our diet. These fatty acids are a certain type in a list of other fatty acids, but this type (omega-3) is the most essential and the most beneficial for our brains and bodies in general. They have numerous effects on the brain, including reducing inflammation (which reduces the risk of Alzheimer's) and maintaining and improving mood and cognitive function, specifically including memory. Omega-3 has these greatly beneficial effects because of the way that it acts in the brain, which is what makes it so essential to our diets. Omega-3 fatty acids increase the production of new nerve cells in the brain by acting specifically on the nerve stem cells within the brain, causing new and healthy nerve cells to be generated.

Omega-3 can be found in fish like salmon, sardines, black cod, and herring. It can also be taken as a pill-form supplement for those who do not eat fish or cannot eat enough of it, as well as a fish oil supplement like krill oil.

Omega-3 fatty acids are by far the most important nutrient that you need to ensure you are ingesting because of the numerous benefits that come from it, both in the brain and in the rest of the body. While supplements are often the last step when it comes to trying to include something in your diet, for omega-3, the benefits are too great to potentially miss by trying to receive all of it from your diet.

Sulforaphane

What do Brussels sprouts, cabbage, kale, and broccoli have in common? All of these green vegetables contain sulforaphane; a plant chemical that is found naturally in these vegetables. It is an antioxidant that acts in a similar way to turmeric and thus has similar benefits. Sulforaphane, like turmeric, induces autophagy in the brain, which helps to reduce the risk of Alzheimer's, Parkinson's, and dementia, which are all neurodegenerative diseases. **Neurodegenerative** means that the cells in the brain called nerves are damaged and broken down, which leads to cognitive decline like Alzheimer's or physical decline as in Parkinson's. These vegetables can help to treat these diseases by slowing their progression, as they are all diseases that come about over time. There is no cure yet, but the treatment at this stage involves delaying the progression of these diseases.

Sulforaphane can be found in the aforementioned vegetables, but the strongest source is in broccoli. It can also be taken concentrated in a supplement form.

Calcium

Calcium is beneficial for the healthy circulation of blood, and for maintaining strong bones and teeth. Calcium can come from dairy products like milk, yogurt, and cheese. It can also be found in leafy greens like kale and broccoli, as well as in fish like sardines.

Magnesium

Magnesium is beneficial for your diet, as it also helps you to maintain strong bones and teeth. Magnesium and calcium are most effective when ingested together, as the former aids in the absorption of the latter. It also helps to reduce migraines and is great for calmness and relieving anxiety. Magnesium can be found in leafy green vegetables like kale and spinach, as well as fruits like bananas and raspberries, legumes like beans and chickpeas, vegetables like peas, cabbage, green beans, asparagus, and Brussels sprouts, and fish like tuna and salmon.

Exogenous Ketones

When tested on animals, even when they were ingested on a normal carbohydrate-intake diet, these exogenous ketones proved to be beneficial in terms of helping with problems like seizures, preventing cancer, anti-inflammation, and anti-anxiety, which are the diseases that we normally see to be assisted by ketosis (which is the state the body enters when it is using fat as a source of fuel instead of carbohydrates).

Electrolytes

When you first begin following an intermittent fasting regime, having electrolyte depletion is quite common. This is because of water weight loss through fat and lower carbohydrate intake, which is often common, as we have discussed. By taking electrolyte supplements, this can help to avoid a deficiency in common electrolytes, like magnesium, potassium, and sodium. Along with this, though, you will need to ensure you are drinking enough water to avoid dehydration.

Iron

This one is a little tricky, but it is worth noting. Iron should be obtained in the right amounts in your diet through whole foods. If you feel like you might be deficient in iron and you are having trouble getting it in the foods you eat, you can visit your doctor for advice on this topic. Iron cannot be supplemented without being referred by a doctor first, as it is something that they would like you to first try to get from your food. If this is becoming a problem, they can give you supplements to take. This is especially a concern if you are not eating much red meat, and this may lead your doctor to want you to begin supplementing. Make an appointment with your doctor to find out more about this topic.

Vitamin D

Vitamin D is found in some foods that have been fortified with it, but in a natural sense, it can be found in only a few foods. These include cheese, fatty fish like salmon and tuna, as well as egg yolks. Another source is mushrooms that have been exposed to UV rays, so the organic ones are likely of this sort.

Vitamin D can be absorbed naturally through sun exposure, so if you live in a sunny place, make sure you get out for some walks or some timer with the sun on your skin. If you live in a colder or gloomier place, consider purchasing a lamp that mimics the sun and provides you with vitamin D in your house. On a sunny day, even if it is cold, going outside and getting sun on your face will give you vitamin D.

This one is something that everyone should be conscious of, but it is especially necessary to examine if you are following a specific diet.

Bioactive Compounds

Bioactive compounds are found within foods and act in the body in beneficial ways. The bioactive compounds found within berries such as acai berries, strawberries, and blueberries are very beneficial for your health. The bioactive compounds in these specific types of berries work in the brain to induce autophagy and reduce inflammation. This leads to the protection of brain cells in this case from oxidative stress. Oxidative stress is something that can happen within the brain when there is an imbalance of oxygen, which can cause reduced cognitive function. These berries and their induction of autophagy help to reduce this by keeping the balance of oxygen at a healthy level.

Importance of Setting Guidelines to be Followed Post-Fast

Research has shown that how and when you break your fast is actually just as important as the fast itself. This part of the fast is known as the re-feedingphase. Because this part of the fast is just as important as the fast itself, ensuring that you have clear guidelines set out for yourself about how you will break your fast is necessary. This will ensure that you can do so in the best way possible, as it may be difficult to think through this type of process with a clear mind after you have just finished fasting for hours. Ensuring that the guidelines are already set out for you will ensure your success post-fast.

If you were to allow yourself to eat whatever you wanted to after your fast, you would likely go straight to the foods that you had been craving all day, and the chances of these being vegetables and lean protein are quite slim. By not setting any guidelines for yourself, you may begin to decide that you need to "reward" yourself at the end of your fast by letting yourself eat anything you like in any amount you like. If there are no guidelines to follow, there is no place to stop, and you may end up in a bingeing cycle of eating too much and then eating nothing and so on. Aside from being unhealthy for you and possibly reversing the progress you made by fasting, this would lead to uncomfortable indigestion and an unhappy gut.

Another reason why setting clear guidelines is important for breaking your fast is that the foods that you turn to in moments of intense hunger and cravings are usually carbohydrate- and calorie-rich foods that do not keep you full for very long. These foods usually do not contain protein, which is the longest-lasting source of energy. Vegetables are also low in calories but high in volume, so they are another good option to ensure you feel satiated and energized without having painful indigestion and a lack of energy.

How to Set Clear Post-Fast Guidelines

Meal planning is extremely beneficial for any sort of diet, as combatting cravings and hunger is often a large part of dieting. Since you know beforehand that you will be dealing with the mental struggles associated with these cravings, it is important to set yourself up for success by taking all decision-making and preparation work out of the equation post-fast. If you were to leave it up to your post-fast self to decide what to eat for dinner, to grocery shop for it, and to prepare it, the chances of saying, *"Whatever, I'm too hungry"*, and ordering a pizza instead are quite high. By having your post-fast meal already portioned and prepared, only needing to be microwaved, you will allow yourself to break your fast in the way you planned without giving yourself the time or space to decide to break the fast in any other way. By making it easier for yourself to microwave a pre-planned meal than to order and wait for a pizza, you know exactly which option you will choose every time.

Another way to set clear guidelines for yourself is to make sure that the foods you know you will crave and reach for will not be easily accessible. If you know that you crave chips and salty snacks and that as soon as you break your fast, you will turn to those, keep those out of the house so that you are unable to eat them even if you wanted to. Keeping only the foods you plan to break your fast with within reach will make it so that you will have no choice but to eat the foods you planned to.

Breaking Your Fast Properly and Carefully

How you break your fast will depend on the time of day at which it occurs and the type of fast that you participated in. In this section, I will go over some general rules fort breaking your fast, but keep in mind that you will need to adjust these slightly to fit your personal fast. The important things to keep in mind are the same among all fasts, however.

Breaking your fast is all about showing your body that you are not undergoing starvation and that there is not going to be an ongoing lack of food, but that it is going to have to get used to eating less often than it used to. After some time, it will adjust to this, but in the beginning, it will be attempting to keep you alive as it thinks that there has been some type of food drought.

There are specific times when it is most important to break your fast in a very deliberate way. These times are closer to the beginning of your introduction of fasting, when you change the duration of fasting if you are working your way up to longer fasts and when you fast for the first time in a while. While it is always important to break your fast with clear guidelines, at these times, it is most important as the chances of experiencing some stomach upset post-fast are the highest. Follow the guidelines below to see what things you should be keeping in mind when you break your fast.

Start with Water

If you are breaking fast in the morning, begin by drinking a glass of water before anything else. This will put something into your stomach and tell your body that it is time to begin working for the day. If you are breaking fast in the evening and have been drinking water all day, stick to water with your meal as you don't want to feed your digestive system too much at once.

Break Fast Slowly

While eating your first meal, you will likely feel the urge to eat very quickly and consume as much as you can, as quickly as you can, as it has been a while since you last ate. It is important to resist this urge as you may experience some bloating or discomfort in the digestion of your food.

Practice mindfulness while eating. This means taking every bite slowly and ensuring that you taste and chew each bite fully. Notice how the food feels in your mouth and how it tastes. Remain in the present moment, focused on the bite you are taking, and try not to think of anything else. Since you have not eaten in a while, try to enjoy the first meal you have after you fast. Instead of eating it so quickly that you don't even remember the taste of it, take your time to savor it.

Things to Watch Out For

If you do decide that fasting is right for you, there may be a time during your fast that you must seek medical advice. Knowing when to seek medical advice and when you may be dealing with regular side-effects of fasting is important to ensure you are fasting in a healthy manner.

Side-effects that signal for you to consult a doctor:

- Nausea

- Dizziness

- Bloody stools

- Vomiting

- Loss of consciousness

- Abdominal or chest pain

If you experience any of the above symptoms while fasting, consult a doctor as there may be some complications or other problems that fasting has brought about.

If you experience diarrhea, this may be caused by a number of things, but more importantly, diarrhea can lead to other more serious issues like dehydration, dizziness, cramping, and malnutrition. If you experience diarrhea while fasting, you can end your fast and see if this clears up through home methods such as hydrating, restoring electrolytes, and consuming potassium-rich foods. If it does, consider trying a different kind of fast or visiting your doctor to determine other, safer ways to fast. However, if you are experiencing severe diarrhea, along with any pains or severe dehydration, contact a doctor immediately.

Tips for staying healthy

Practice indeed makes perfect. To help you get into intermittent fasting, I have outlined a few down-to-earth routes and hands-on tips to guide you. Your approach to fasting can mean the difference between success and failure. So, consider these tips as guidelines that will help you to safely implement your preferred fasting regimen.

Find a Worthy Goal

First things first, find a goal that is worth pursuing, or else you will drop the idea at the first hurdle. If you don't have a goal that represents a strong ideal, it won't be long before you start telling yourself, "*I think I've passed the stage of such childishness.*" And yes, many people start a new lifestyle change for reasons that they can't keep up when things get tough. For example, the desire to look like models on TV, or social media making losing weight feel like a social necessity; some trends can be harmful. These reasons are not enough to keep anyone committed to a full lifestyle change and few wonder why so many people with goals are quick to jump from one lifestyle to another.

Don't go into fasting intermittently because it is the thing to do at the moment. Instead, look for inspiring goals, such as:

- Staying fit, young, and healthy.

- Improving your cognitive functions.

- Improving your overall vitality and increasing energy levels.

- Balancing hormones, especially during menopausal or post-menopausal stages of life.

- Improving your overall health, thereby increasing longevity.

Do any of these sound good to you? Surely at this stage of your life, you are aware of the inherent risks of doing something merely because others are doing it too. That type of motivation will fail you.

Check Your Hormones

A woman's hormones can be affected by changes in her patterns of behavior. Whether it is a physical change, such as altering their eating pattern, or an emotional change, such as being irritated or sad, it can bring about hormonal imbalances, even temporarily.

But for perimenopausal and menopausal women, hormones can go haywire for reasons even they can't define. She could be feeling really great all week, and without anything changing, she could suddenly become fatigued, depressed, and not in the right frame of mind. These changes happen due to the unpredictability of this phase of a woman's life. Because this can happen for no apparent reason, it is best to check your hormonal levels before putting your body through any major lifestyle changes. If you've ever had issues with thyroid, cortisol, or adrenal fatigue, ensure that you have these checked before you begin.

This may come as a surprise to some women, but your ovaries produce testosterone too. So, as you grow older and begin to experience a decline in your estrogen and progesterone levels, your testosterone levels are also taking a nosedive. Your libido can be affected by low levels of testosterone and make you feel exhausted for no reason at all. While you are checking your other hormones, don't forget to do a testosterone test. The thyroid and testosterone hormones also help in weight regulation. So, if you intend to shed some weight using intermittent fasting, these tests are very necessary.

Start Slow

To go from having five or six meals daily to eating only once a day can lead to very dire consequences. In addition to being harmful to your health, massive and abrupt changes are hardly sustainable. After confirming that intermittent fasting is suitable for your health, the next thing to do is plan how to ease into the habit. Take another look at the example of how to ease into fasting in Chapter 2 and consider following it or coming up with something similar that works for you. In other words, before you fully implement any intermittent fasting regimen, it is a good practice to first test the waters, so to speak, with a less strict form of fasting. By doing this, it will help your body acclimate to the changes before going into the proper regimen.

Don't Fuss Over What You Can Eat

One common mistake people make when fasting is obsessing over the fasting hours and what to eat when they are finally allowed. You don't have to worry about if you are fasting as long as someone else, the important thing is what's comfortable for you. Of course, if your fasting window is too small, you are not likely to see any results. Also, don't get too tied up in every little detail of intermittent fasting. For example, you don't have to become too worried because you missed a day. Remember that fasting intermittently should be a lifestyle change if you want to continue to reap the benefits. And for a lifestyle change to be sustainable, you must be able to adapt in the face of challenges. Missing a day or cutting your fast short for reasons beyond your control shouldn't get you worked up and worrying about whether you can do the entire plan. Don't give up.

Again, some people focus too much on what they can or cannot eat. For example, "*Can I add just a little butter or cream?*", "*Would it hurt to eat this type of food during the fasting window?*" If your focus is on what you can have while you are fasting, you are giving your attention to the wrong things and putting your mind in an unhelpful state. Give your mind the right focus by concentrating on doing a good, clean fast, and try to consume only water, tea, or coffee during the window.

Watch Electrolytes

Your body's electrolytes are compounds and elements that occur naturally in body fluids, blood, and urine. They can also be ingested through drinks, foods, and supplements. Some of them include magnesium, calcium, potassium, chloride, phosphate, and sodium. Their functions include fluid balance, regulation of heart and neurological functions, acid-base balance, oxygen delivery, and many other functions.

It is important to keep these electrolytes in a state of balance, but many people who practice fasting tend to neglect this and run into problems. Here is a common notion: "Don't let anything into your stomach until the end of your fast." Even those just starting to fast know it doesn't work that way, and they tend to forget or fully stay away from liquids during their fasting window.

When you lose too much water from your body through sweating, vomiting, and diarrhea, or you don't have enough water in your body because you don't drink enough liquids, you increase the risk of electrolyte disorders. It is not okay to drink tea or black coffee throughout the morning period of your fast window. You will wear yourself down if you don't drink enough water. The longer you fast without water, the higher your chances of flushing out electrolytes and running into trouble. You can end up raising your blood pressure, developing muscle twitching and spasms, fatigue, fast or irregular heartbeat, and many other health problems.

On the other hand, drinking too much water can also tip the water-electrolyte balance. What you want to do is to drink adequate amounts of water and not excess, whether you are fasting or not.

Give the Calorie Restriction a Rest

Remember that intermittent fasting is different from dieting. Your focus should be on eating healthily during your eating windows or days instead of focusing on calorie restriction. Even if you are fasting for weight loss, don't obsess over calories. Following a fasting regimen is enough to take care of the calories you consume. It is absolutely unnecessary to engage in a practice that can hurt your metabolism. Combining intermittent fasting with eating too little food in your eating window because you are worried about your calorie intake can cause problems for your metabolism.

One of the major reasons that people push themselves into restricting calories while fasting is their concern for rapid weight loss. You need to be wary of any process that brings about drastic physical changes to your body in very short amounts of time. While it is okay to desire quick results, your health and safety are more important. When you obsess or worry that you are not losing weight as quickly as you want, you are not helping matters. Instead, you are increasing your stress level, which is counterproductive. You are already taking practical steps toward losing weight by intermittent fasting; why would you want to undo your hard work by unnecessary worrying?

Simply focus on following a sustainable intermittent fasting regimen and let go of the need to restrict your calorie intake. Intermittent fasting will give your body the right number of calories it needs if you do it properly.

The First Meal of the Eating Window Is Key

Breaking your fast is a crucial part of the process because, if you don't get it right, it could quickly develop into unhealthy eating patterns. When you break your fast, it is important to have healthy foods around to prevent grabbing unhealthy, feel-good snacks. Make sure what you are eating in your window is not a high-sugar or high-carb meal. I recommend that you consider breaking your fast with something that is highly nutritious such as a green smoothie, protein shake, or healthy salad.

As much as possible, avoid breaking your fast with foods from a fast-food restaurant. Eating junk food after your fast is a quick way to ruin all the hard work you've put in during your fasting window. If, for any reason, you can't prepare your meal, ensure that you order very specific foods that will complement your effort and not destroy what you've built.

Break Your Fast Gently

It is okay to feel very hungry after going a long time without food, even if you were drinking water all through the fasting window. This is particularly true for people who are just starting fasting. But don't let the intensity of your hunger push you to eat. You don't want to force food hurriedly into your stomach after going long without food, or you might hurt yourself and experience stomach distress. Take it slow when you break your fast; eat light meals in small portions initially. Wait for a couple of minutes for your stomach to get used to the presence of food again before continuing with a normal-sized meal. The waiting period will douse any hunger pangs and remove the urge to rush your meal. For example, break your fast with a small serving of salad and wait for about 15 minutes. Drink some water and then after about five more minutes, you can eat a normal-sized meal.

Nutrition is Important

Although intermittent fasting is not dieting and so does not specify which foods to eat, limit, and completely avoid, it makes sense to eat healthily. This means focusing on eating a balanced diet, such as:

1. Whole grains.

2. Fruits and vegetables (canned in water, fresh, or frozen).

3. Lean sources of protein (lentils, beans, eggs, poultry, tofu, and so on).

4. Healthy fats (nuts, seeds, coconuts, avocados, olive oil, olive, and fatty fish).

It simply doesn't make any sense to go for 16 hours (or more) without food and then spend the rest of the day eating junk. Even if you follow the 5:2 diet and limit your calorie intake to only 500 calories per day for two days, it is totally illogical to follow it with five days of eating highly processed foods and low-quality meals. Combining intermittent fasting with unbalanced diets will lead to nutritional deficiencies and defeat the goal of fasting in the first place. Realize that intermittent fasting is not a magic wand that makes all poor eating habits vanish in a poof. For the practice to work, you must be deliberate about the types of food you eat.

Find a Regimen That Works for You

Don't follow a fasting diet because it seems to suit someone else. Instead, go for something that fits into your schedule. If you feel caged or boxed in by a particular fasting plan, it is a clear indication that it is not a suitable plan for you. Thankfully, you have the freedom to design something that works for you, even if you are following a specific regimen. The regimens are not carved in stone; they are flexible, and you can adjust them to suit you as long as you follow each regimen's basic principles. For example, if you decide to follow the 16:8 fasting regimen, your 8-hour eating window must not strictly be between noon and 8pm. You have the option of tailoring the eating window to something that gives you room to handle other aspects of your life, such as work, hobbies, family, and so on. You might decide to make your 8-hour eating window from 9am to 5pm, or from 1pm to 9pm.

Whatever you choose to do is totally up to you. After all, it is your life, and you have the freedom to choose what you want. Books, the internet, and even loved ones can only suggest and offer recommendations. Ultimately, the final decision rests with you. Since your goal is not to please someone else or seek external approval, you should make your choice based on what is most convenient for you. You are seeking results, not accolades. Therefore, don't follow something unrealistic or too restrictive for you. Even if you endure the most stringent type of fast and get admiration and commendation from others, have you considered what that fasting regimen is doing to your overall health? The body is delicately designed, and putting it through unnecessary stress is unsafe if you are merely enduring discomfort to boost your ego.

Conclusion

Thank you for reading to the end of this book! I hope that, through the pages of this book, you were able to gain the knowledge, understanding, and confidence you need to succeed with losing weight and improving your health.

While intermittent fasting may be an unorthodox lifestyle at this point, for centuries, it was a standard and everyday part of life worldwide. Not only that, but science has proven it to be both safe and effective. There is no reason to hold back from this positive lifestyle that has proven through both time and science to be such an improvement. You have everything to gain and nothing to lose by taking a step forward and making a change for the better. Whether you choose to practice intermittent fasting alone or with the ketogenic diet, you can expect to experience many benefits. While it may take a little time to adjust to the change in lifestyle, as all changes do, take heart in knowing that within a month, most people adjust and adapt.

CPSIA information can be obtained
at www.ICGtesting.com
Printed in the USA
BVHW091938060521
606647BV00006B/1054

9 781802 742039